WHAT TO DO
WHEN YOUR CHILD GETS SICK

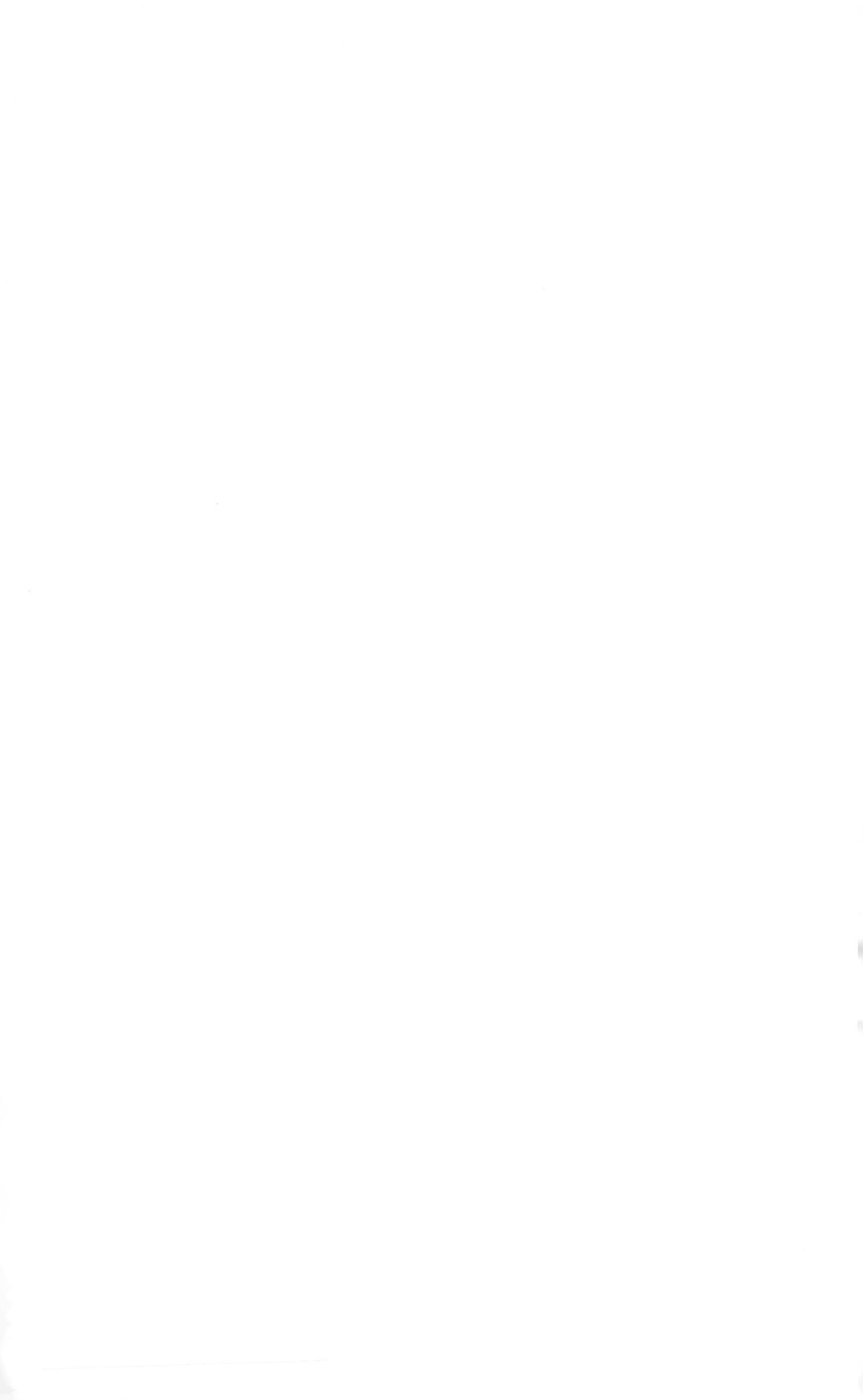

WHAT TO DO WHEN YOUR CHILD GETS SICK

THE ESSENTIAL EMERGENCY MANUAL FOR PARENTS AND CARERS

Associate Professor Paul Middleton,
Dr Andrew Ratchford,
Dr John Mackenzie
& Dr Jason Smith

ARENA
ALLEN&UNWIN

Arena Books, an imprint of
Allen & Unwin
83 Alexander Street
Crows Nest NSW 2065
Australia
Phone: (61 2) 8425 0100
Fax: (61 2) 9906 2218
Email: info@allenandunwin.com
Web: www.allenandunwin.com

Cataloguing-in-Publication details are available
from the National Library of Australia
www.librariesaustralia.nla.gov.au

ISBN 978 1 74175 686 9

Internal design by Emily O'Neill
Illustrations by Melinda Klinger
Index by Russell Brooks
Set in 12/15 pt Bembo by Mary Trewby and by Midland Typesetters, Australia
Printed in China at Everbest Printing Co

10 9 8 7 6 5 4 3 2 1

Associate Professor Paul Middleton is an emergency doctor with extensive experience with sick children. He has worked in major hospitals in Australia and the UK and was part of retrieval teams with CareFlight and Westpac rescue helicopters. He has taught hundreds of doctors and nurses how to treat serious childhood illness and injury as a paediatric life support instructor. He is Senior Medical Adviser to the Ambulance Service of NSW and Chair of the NSW branch of the Australian Resuscitation Council. He has two young children.

Dr Andrew Ratchford is an Emergency Physician and Clinical Lecturer in Medicine at the University of Sydney. He has worked for the London Helicopter Emergency Service, treating critically injured adults and children. He has attended sick children for more than 15 years and teaches paediatric life support courses to doctors, nurses and paramedics in Australia, the UK, Cambodia and Fiji.

Dr John Mackenzie works at a busy emergency department in NSW, treating sick children every day. He is a medical advisor to the Ambulance Service of NSW. He spent two years in Africa with Médecins Sans Frontières, has been a General Practitioner in New Zealand and was part of a medical retrieval team with the Westpac and Surf Lifesaving rescue helicopter services. He has two young children.

Dr Jason Smith is a consultant in emergency medicine in the UK. He undertook specialist training in emergency medicine and is a Senior Lecturer in Pre-Hospital and Emergency Medicine. He has had extensive clinical experience with paediatric emergencies in the UK and in challenging environments overseas. Jason has three children of his own.

CONTENTS

INTRODUCTION

It is almost inconceivable that children are dying from something that starts as a fever or asthma. However, every day in every country thousands of children are rushed into emergency departments, many critically ill, because nobody realised how sick they were becoming.

Dr Paul Middleton has seen too many children come through hospital doors when it is too late for life-saving treatment. It is heart-breaking for doctors and nurses, but even worse for parents, who are left wondering whether they could have done something sooner, could have seen the signs earlier? This motivated Paul and three other emergency specialists to write *What to Do When Your Child Gets Sick* and teach parents and people who care for children how to recognise the key signs that a child is becoming seriously ill.

Even with CPR, very few children survive because they have been too ill, for too long. The key to saving children is to never get to this point; there is a window of opportunity before they rapidly deteriorate. We want to teach parents and carers how to stop their child from dying of preventable causes.

Do *you* know:

- when noisy breathing in a child is dangerous?
- what breathing recession is?
- how to assess a child's level of consciousness?
- how to perform a simple glass test to recognise a meningococcal rash?
- when a fever is manageable at home or when it is life-threatening?

In the middle of the night at home, when your child is sick or when they are at day-care or when grandparents are babysitting, it is unlikely a nurse or doctor will be on hand.

What to Do When Your Child Gets Sick aims to give you the information you'll need for any medical emergency you might face with your child, or a child in your care. It also covers a wide range of less serious – but nonetheless frightening – medical conditions, such as the management of broken bones, seizures (fits) and burns. This book is a vital source of information for people looking after children – including parents, teachers, babysitters, day-care and preschool staff, and nannies.

The book is divided into four sections:

Part I: Understanding the Body – an overview of how the body works

Part II: Your Unwell Child – how to recognise if your child is ill and what to do

Part III: Your Injured Child – accidents and injuries that may happen and what to do

Part IV: Essentials – vital information about first aid and what to do in an emergency.

Children do not have a cardiac arrest for the same reasons as adults – so it is often difficult to judge when a child is becoming so ill that they may have a cardiac arrest. Fortunately, reversing the problems that lead to cardiac arrest in children is often relatively straightforward, and includes ensuring that they can get enough oxygen and fluid.

At the end of the chapters in Parts II and III about illnesses and injuries are easy-to-use flowcharts that allow you to quickly access the essentials of what to do if your child is unwell. These will help you recognise if your child is very sick and whether you need to take them to your GP, to a hospital emergency department or call an ambulance. Within each of these chapters there is general advice on how to manage less serious medical problems at home.

This book uses the best up-to-date medical information, and has been written by emergency specialists who see and treat sick children every day and are involved in teaching these principles to medical, nursing and allied health personnel on a regular basis.

Nurses and doctors in hospitals, and paramedics out of hospital, are trained to the highest standards, through courses provided by bodies such as the Australian Resuscitation Council and the Royal Australasian College of Surgeons, to recognise and manage seriously ill and injured patients. In *What to Do When Your Child Gets Sick* we teach parents, carers and the public what we teach doctors, nurses and paramedics – specifically to recognise both potential and serious illness and injury in children, and what to do about it.

The authors run a course called Saving LittleLives, which teaches parents and carers how to recognise the signs that a child is becoming seriously ill. For more information go to <www.savinglittlelives.com>.

PART I

Understanding the Body

This part of the book is all about understanding how your child's body works. Chapter 1, How the body works, looks at the normal body functions (physiology) and normal body structure (anatomy) of children. Chapter 2, Size matters, explains how the structure and function of children's bodies differ from that of adults, and also the differences between babies, small children and older children. In Chapter 3, Growing up, the normal changes you can expect as your child grows are described.

All the information in these chapters will help you to understand what's normal and how to recognise changes that may occur when your child is ill or injured. It is also helpful to understand how the different systems of the body are affected by injury and illness. A basic knowledge of how your child's body works normally is essential to allow you to understand what happens when they are sick.

1

HOW THE BODY WORKS

To recognise and treat childhood illness and injury you need to understand how they affect the systems of the body. A basic knowledge of how the body works normally is essential to understanding an abnormal situation. This chapter teaches you about basic anatomy and physiology, in particular the 'ABC' of life support – Airway, Breathing and Circulation. The respiratory system (airway and breathing), the cardiovascular system (circulation) and the all-important immune system are discussed in detail, along with an overview of the other systems in the body and how they work.

Put simply, physiology is the study of how living things work and function and anatomy is the structure and the parts of your body. Anatomy and physiology are what make you a living, breathing, walking and talking human being. They are both vast subjects, numerous books have been written about them, and we won't attempt to cover them in any great depth here; however, you do need a basic understanding of how your heart and lungs work to keep you alive.

COMPOSITION OF THE BODY

Your body is composed of cells, tissues, organs and systems.

Cells These tiny, living particles form the basic building blocks of all your body tissues and organs.

Tissues These are more complex than cells but are made up of many similar cells joined together by other non-living substances. Examples of tissues are your muscles and bones.

Organs More complex again than tissues, organs are made up of several different types of tissue and they perform a specific function. For example, the heart is made up of muscle, blood vessels and nerves (all separate tissues) and it has the specific function of pumping blood around the body.

Systems The most complex of the structures in the body, they are the many different organs and tissues which perform vital functions in the body. The respiratory system, for example, comprises the airways (mouth, nose, throat, windpipe), lungs, blood vessels, lymphatic tissues, chest wall (bones and muscles) and diaphragm (a strong muscle), with the specific function of taking oxygen from the air and converting it into oxygen in the blood.

Your body is made up of various types of tissue (such as muscle, bone, skin and nerves). All these tissues are composed of tiny individual particles known as cells. Most cells have a control centre, or nucleus, containing your DNA – the basic template from which your body is designed and built.

Cells require a constant source of energy to survive. Energy is made when different types of foods – carbohydrates, fats and protein – break down inside the body with the aid of oxygen (a process known as aerobic metabolism). Oxygen is a major component of the

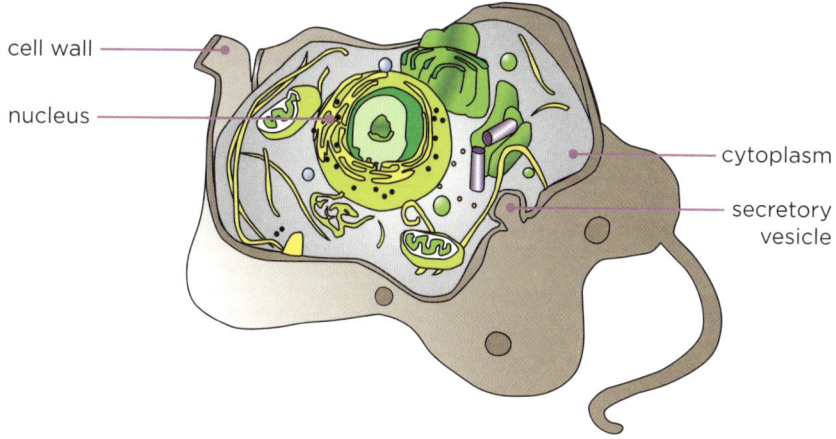

cell wall

nucleus

cytoplasm

secretory vesicle

Diagram of a typical body cell showing the components. The nucleus is the control centre in the middle of the cell and contains DNA, the cell's hereditary material that directs the cell to perform specific functions in the body.

air we breathe in; what we breathe out is the waste product from this process, carbon dioxide.

If the supply of oxygen is interrupted, or if the demand by the body is too high, energy may be created in the absence of oxygen (a process known as anaerobic metabolism), but this is much less efficient and can only be maintained for short periods. Cells that do not get enough oxygen will eventually die – therefore, the constant supply of oxygen is paramount. The cells that make up your vital organs – brain, heart, lungs and kidneys – will begin to die after only three to four minutes if the oxygen supply is cut off. This is why the most important factor in the maintenance of life is the supply of oxygen.

The uptake of oxygen and the elimination of carbon dioxide by your body are achieved by breathing (respiration). Respiration can be divided into two types: external and internal.

External respiration is the process of you using your lungs and chest wall to breathe, and this allows oxygen to move from the lungs into your blood stream.

Internal respiration is when gas (oxygen) is exchanged between your blood and the cells of your body. The work of transporting oxygen to your body's organs is done by your cardiovascular system – your heart and blood vessels. The cardiovascular system also transports waste products, such as carbon dioxide, from your organs to your lungs, which you then expel through breathing out.

Your respiratory system comprises the structures involved in removing oxygen from the air you breathe (external respiration), and the individual cells and blood vessels that transfer the oxygen to your organs and tissues (internal respiration). The cardiovascular system, also known as the circulatory system, comprises the heart and the blood vessels and has the vital role of pumping blood (containing oxygen) to your body. Your body's ability to resist infections is done by your immune system. But before we move on to these three in more detail, it is good to be aware of the other systems of your body.

The lungs inside the chest are supplied with air through the trachea. The air then passes into the different lobes of both lungs via the bronchi. The diaphragm is the strong flat sheet of muscle that separates the chest from the abdomen and helps with breathing.

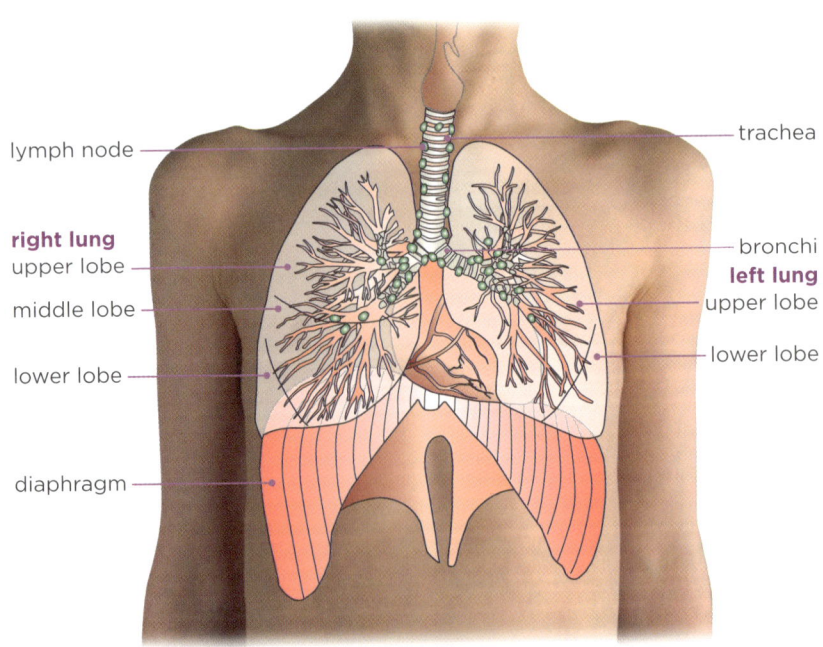

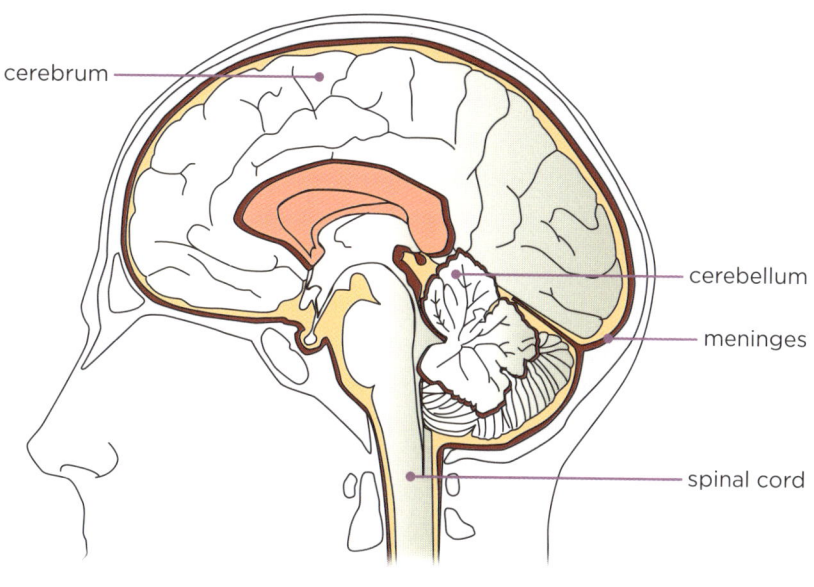

cerebrum

cerebellum

meninges

spinal cord

The brain is encased in the bony skull and covered by three protective layers called the meninges. The left and right sides of the brain, or cerebrum, are the thinking part of the brain and also store memories and produce language. The cerebellum is connected to the parts of the brain that control movements and sensations.

THE NERVOUS SYSTEM

Consisting of the brain, spinal cord and nerves, your nervous system controls all the other systems in your body, and it is also responsible for your thoughts, memory and personality. It controls communication between your different body systems and between you and the outside world.

THE DIGESTIVE SYSTEM

This is responsible for breaking food down into individual molecules or particles so that it can be used by the different cells in your body for energy. The digestive system consists of your gastrointestinal tract (or alimentary canal) and other supporting tissues and organs. The gastrointestinal tract starts at your mouth and finishes at the anus,

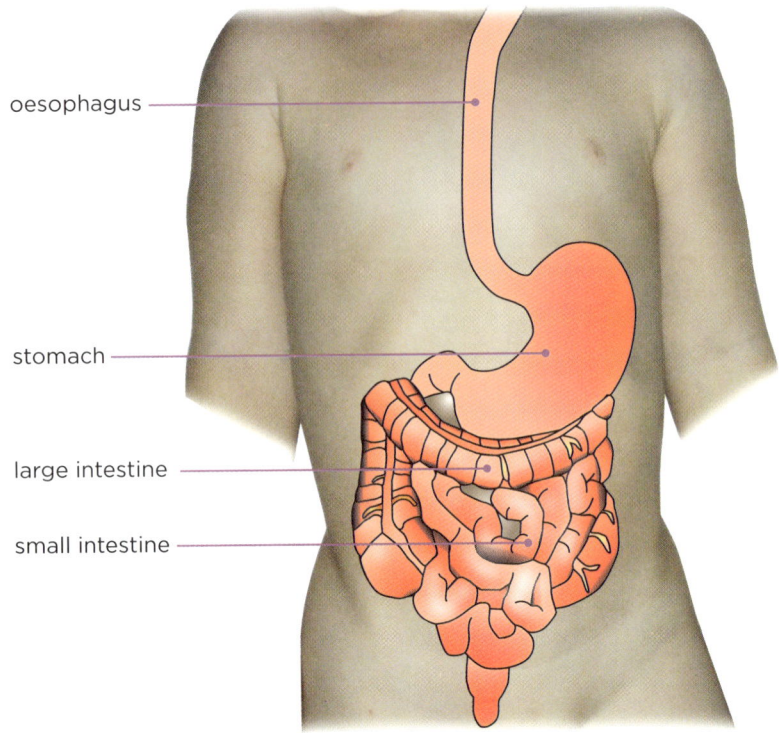

The gastrointestinal tract is divided into two parts. Food travels through the oesophagus and stomach in the upper gastrointestinal tract to the lower tract, where it is broken down in the intestines. Energy and nutrients are extracted and the remaining matter is expelled through the anus.

and is made up of mouth, tongue, teeth, oesophagus (or food pipe), stomach, small intestine and large intestine. Digestion (the process of breaking food into molecules) is helped by fluids secreted into the gastrointestinal tract from salivary glands in the mouth, and from the liver, gall bladder and pancreas.

THE GENITOURINARY SYSTEM

The genitourinary system comprises two different systems – your reproductive system and your urinary system. The main function of the reproductive system is, of course, to produce offspring for the survival of the species. For women, it is the production and fertilisation

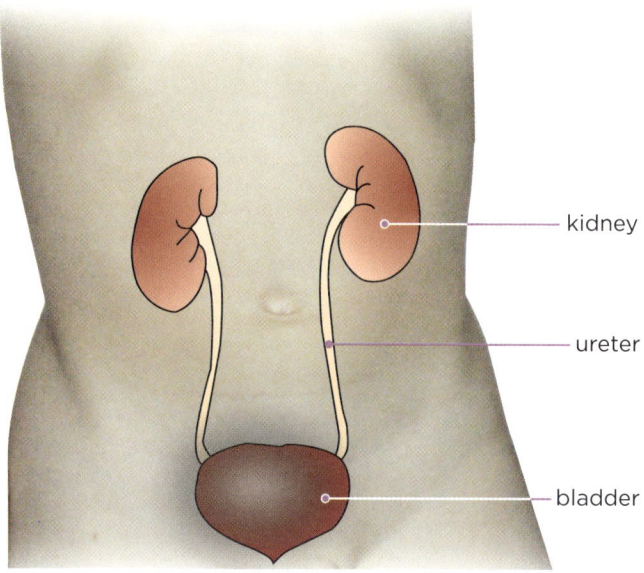

The kidneys, positioned near the middle of the back, clean the blood by filtering out waste products and turning them into urine. This passes through the ureters into the bladder, where it is stored until expelled by urination.

of egg cells and the nurturing environment for the development of a foetus. For men, this includes the production of sperm cells and how these are delivered to the female.

The urinary system controls the amount of liquids and essential salts in your body, and also the excretion of unwanted waste products of internal respiration occurring in the cells. The urinary system is made up of the two kidneys, ureters, bladder and the urethra, which carries urine to the outside.

THE LYMPHATIC SYSTEM

There are three main functions of the lymphatic system, the most important being the fight against infection (this is described in more detail in 'The immune system', page 30). Its other functions are to help remove tiny fat particles from your digestive tract, and to remove excess fluid from your tissues and return it to the blood.

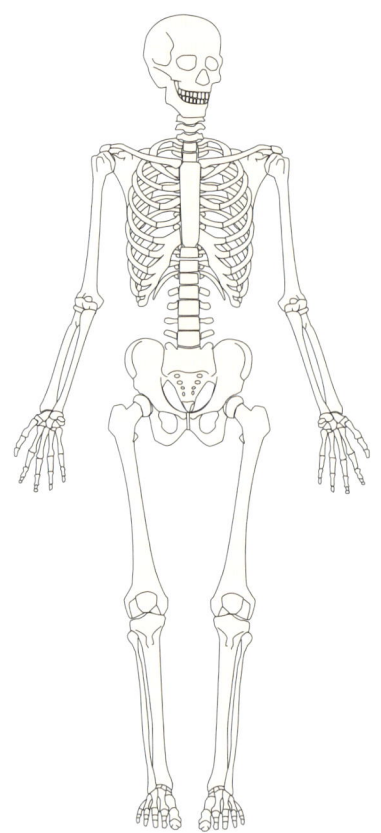

The bony skeleton. The bones are connected by joints and held together by the muscular system.

THE MUSCULOSKELETAL SYSTEM

The structure of the body mainly comprises bones (your skeleton or skeletal system) and muscles (your muscular system). These allow you to walk, talk and breathe but also have some protective properties; for example, the ribs protect the lungs and heart and the skull protects the brain.

THE RESPIRATORY SYSTEM
'A' is for 'airway'

The airway is the part of your body that allows air into your lungs. It starts at your nose and the mouth, and passes the back of your throat to your windpipe (or trachea). From there it descends into your chest to connect to the lungs.

Your nose consists of your nostrils and the much larger internal cavity. The surface of the internal cavity is made of soft tissue called mucous membrane, which is composed of folds and has a very good blood supply close to the surface (this is why nose bleeds are so common). The blood in the folded lining warms and humidifies air as it passes through the nose, and the folds also filter large particles before they pass into the lungs. If the nose is blocked, by injury or swelling of the mucous membranes (as when you have a cold or allergic reaction), you tend to breathe more through your mouth.

At the back of the throat, the passages from the nose and mouth meet to form the pharynx. This area is where your tonsils lie. The tonsils are small organs that contain lymphoid tissue, part of the immune system, which protects our bodies from infection. When infected, lymphoid tissue swells the surrounding area as it filters the blood containing the infecting organisms (bacteria or viruses). In severe infection, the swelling may be enough to cause airway blockage.

The lower part of the pharynx divides into two pathways. The trachea (windpipe) leads to the lungs and the oesophagus (gullet) leads to the stomach. At the top of the trachea is the larynx (or voice box), the front part of which, the thyroid cartilage, can be felt and is known as the 'Adam's apple'. Usually solid and liquid material entering the pharynx is channelled down the oesophagus by a flap

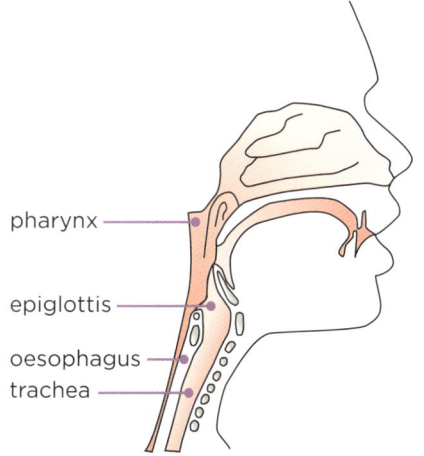

pharynx

epiglottis

oesophagus

trachea

A cross-section of the mouth and throat, showing the pharynx, trachea (windpipe) and oesophagus (gullet). To prevent choking, a flap of tissue called the epiglottis covers the windpipe whenever food is swallowed.

of tissue called the epiglottis. This flips over and covers the opening to the larynx during swallowing, but the opening lies open during normal breathing. When a bit of food 'goes down the wrong way' it is because this protective mechanism has failed and food enters the larynx, causing the cough reflex. If the cough reflex fails to remove the piece of foreign material, choking occurs.

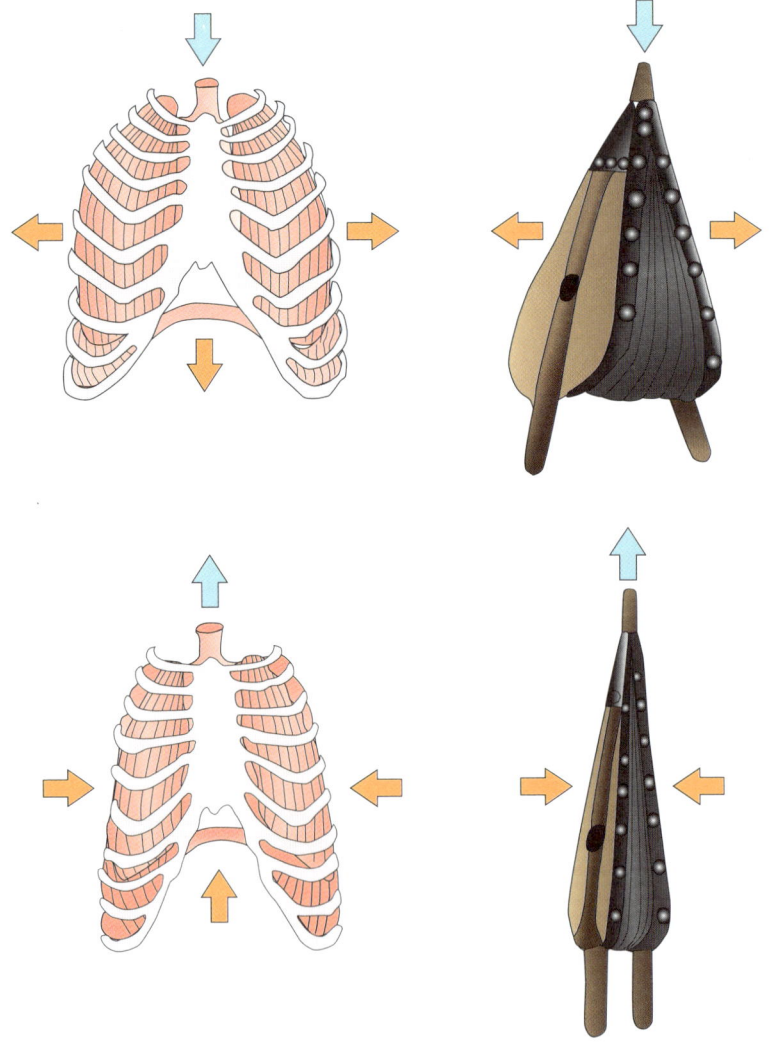

As the muscles of the chest pull the ribs up and out, the lungs are pulled open, sucking in air. As the chest muscles relax, the air is forced out of the lungs again.

'B' is for 'breathing'

Your lungs sit inside the chest cavity, like a pair of partially deflated balloons inside a pair of bellows. In order to draw air into your lungs, the chest wall must expand outwards and upwards, making your chest larger and pulling the walls of the balloons apart, sucking air in. This is called inspiration and it is achieved during normal breathing by the contraction of muscles called the intercostal muscles, which lie between your ribs. This lifts the ribcage up and out. In heavier breathing, extra power for inspiration is achieved by the contraction of the diaphragmatic muscles, which pull the diaphragm (the strong flat muscle sheet that separates the abdomen and the chest) down.

Both of these processes result in the inflation of the chest, but in some disease situations use of other muscles to aid breathing is a sign of respiratory distress, especially in children. This is an important concept that will be discussed later (see Breathing, page 34).

In expiration (when you breathe out) all the respiratory muscles relax, allowing the natural elasticity of the lungs to pull your chest wall inwards, forcing air out. It is possible to aid this passive process by contracting the intercostal muscles and thereby pulling the ribs in harder, forcing breath out, as when you blow out a candle. When resting, an adult only moves about half a litre of air in and out with each breath (the tidal volume), although the lungs may hold a total of up to 6 litres. (Children's lungs are always smaller and therefore hold a smaller amount of air. The size of their lungs is related to the size of their body, increasing as they get older.) During exercise, the tidal volume increases to support the body's increased demand for oxygen.

Your trachea is the airway pipe that leads from the larynx to the lungs and it is held open and supported by rings of cartilage, which is

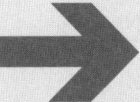

DANGER SIGNS
As children become more ill and exhausted, the earlier signs of fast breathing and chest recession may disappear. This does not mean that they are getting better, but rather that they are becoming gravely ill and need immediate treatment.

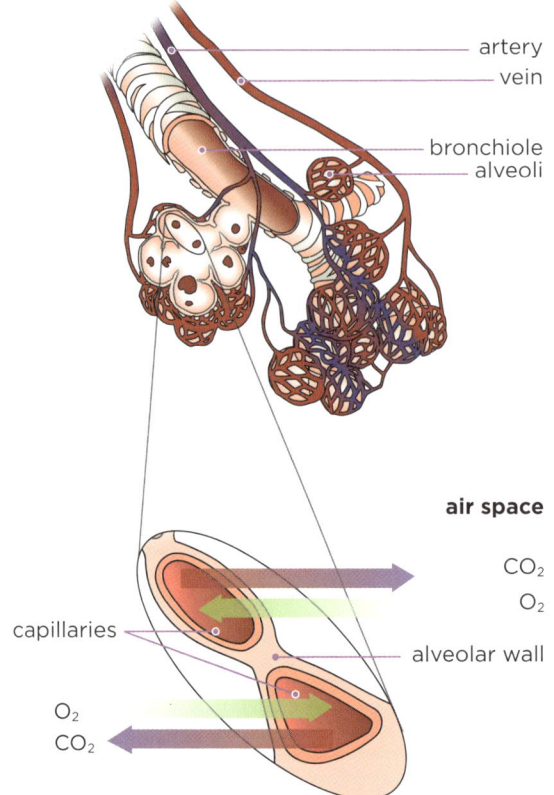

artery
vein
bronchiole
alveoli

air space

CO_2
O_2

capillaries

alveolar wall

O_2
CO_2

The smallest air passages in the lungs end in tiny air sacs, or alveoli, which are the body's primary gas exchange units. The alveoli move incoming oxygen from the air into the blood and waste products (carbon dioxide) from the blood back into the lungs, from where they are exhaled through the mouth and the nose.

a firm but flexible support tissue. After entering the chest cavity the trachea splits into two main bronchi, one supplying each lung. Your two lungs are made up of several separate sections, or lobes. The two large bronchi further divide into smaller bronchi, one supplying each lobe of the lung, then into even smaller pipes called bronchioles. This is the point where the pipes lose their cartilage support.

The pipes carry on dividing like branches of a tree, and their size (diameter) reduces with each division until the smallest of the bronchioles ends in tiny air sacs in the lungs, called alveoli. The walls of these alveoli are only one cell thick, and are surrounded by the smallest blood vessels of the lung, the capillaries. The walls of these capillaries are also only one cell thick and this is where gas exchange takes place. Oxygen enters the blood from the alveoli and waste carbon dioxide is released back into the lungs for disposal.

How we use oxygen

The blood that arrives in the lungs from the rest of your body is venous blood (the blood in the veins). This blood is relatively low in oxygen and high in carbon dioxide. As it passes through your lungs, it takes up oxygen from the alveoli and releases carbon dioxide (the process known as internal respiration). By the time the blood leaves the lung via your arteries (now called arterial blood) it is high in oxygen and low in carbon dioxide. Arterial blood then carries oxygen to the rest of your body.

The opposite of this happens when blood reaches the organs and tissues in your body. The oxygen from the blood moves into the cells, which use it to burn fuel for energy. The waste products of the process (carbon dioxide) are released back into the blood to be carried back to the lungs in the veins, and the process is repeated.

Oxygen carried in your blood is attached to a protein called haemoglobin, which is inside the red blood cells. Haemoglobin picks up oxygen in the lungs and carries it around your body, releasing it for uptake by the tissues. Haemoglobin, when carrying oxygen, is bright red in colour, making this the colour of arterial blood, but when it is not carrying oxygen it is darker, which is why venous blood is darker in colour than arterial blood.

THE CARDIOVASCULAR SYSTEM

Your heart is the centre of all this blood movement. It is located in the middle of your chest cavity, in between your lungs, and bulges farther to the left. It is made up of two sides, the right and the left, and each side is split into two chambers.

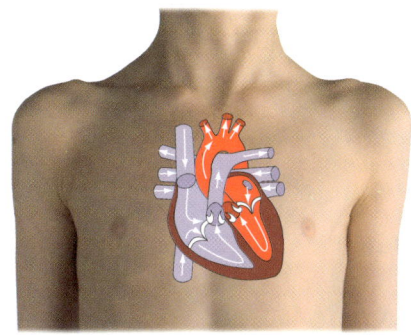

The heart lies behind the sternum, or breastbone, with its main part usually slightly to the left of centre.

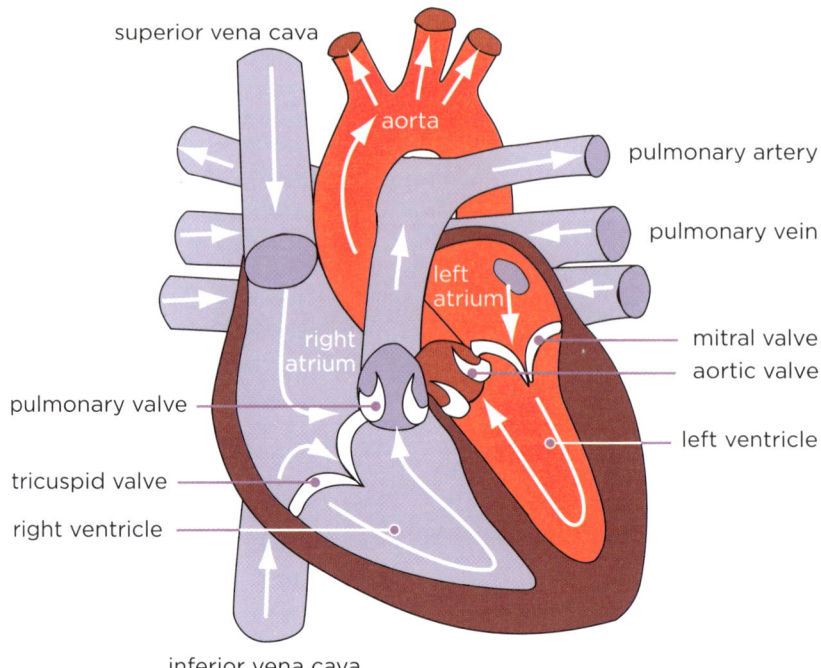

Cross-section of the heart with arrows indicating the flow of blood. In the human body, the heart operates as a double-circulatory system, with two separate pumping mechanisms and four chambers (two atriums, two ventricles). De-oxygenated blood is collected in the right atrium and pumped, via the right ventricle, into the lungs. There carbon dioxide is filtered out and oxygen added. The oxygenated blood then flows into the left atrium, where it is pumped, via the left ventricle, through the body.

Blood coming through your veins from the body's peripheral organs enters the right side of your heart. From there it is pumped by the heart to your lungs, where it picks up oxygen and gets rid of carbon dioxide. When blood leaves your lungs it passes into the left side of your heart from where, full of oxygen once again, it is pumped around your body through your arteries. Arterial blood leaves your heart at a high pressure. The blood returning to the heart is travelling in the lower pressure system of your veins.

Between the arteries and veins, inside the peripheral tissues, blood passes through tiny blood vessels called capillaries, where gas exchange occurs.

Pumping blood around the body

The heart is made up of special muscle tissue which, unlike any other muscle, contracts spontaneously and rhythmically without external stimulation. This happens because there are electrical impulses that originate in the heart muscle, usually at special areas called natural pacemakers. When an adult is resting, the rate at which their heart produces these electrical impulses to stimulate contraction is usually between 60 to 100 heartbeats per minute, but drugs and the nervous

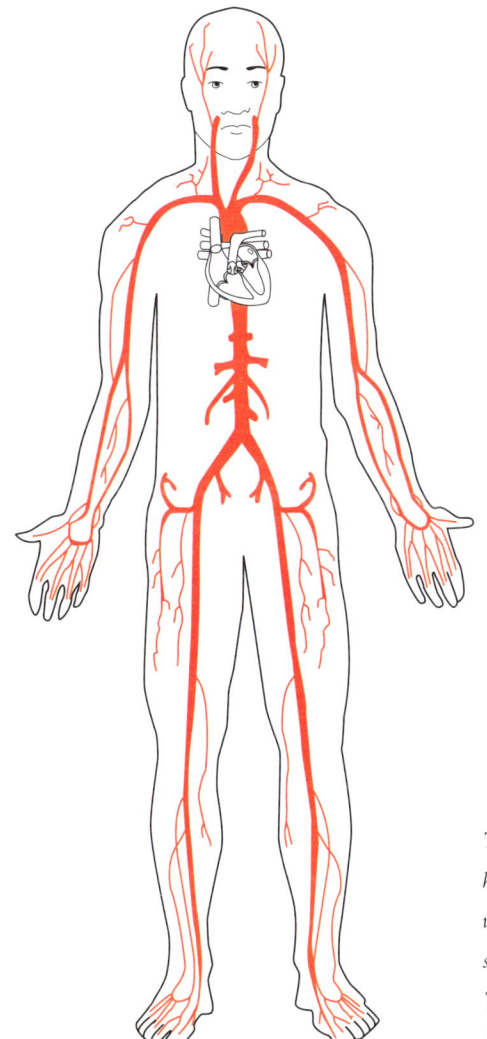

The oxygenated blood pumped out of the heart is carried around the body in the arteries, which are a major part of the circulatory system. Arterial blood is high in oxygen. The blood flowing into the heart is called 'venous' blood.

system can influence this. For example, adrenaline, a naturally occurring drug produced by the body in response to shock, speeds up the heart.

The heart acts as a pump, going through a cycle of contraction and relaxation. At the height of contraction the pressure inside the arteries is at its highest, called the systolic blood pressure. As the heart relaxes the pressure in the arteries falls, until it reaches the lowest pressure, called the diastolic blood pressure. When your blood pressure is taken the ratio between the systolic (when the heart is contracted) pressure and the diastolic (when the heart is relaxed) pressure is measured. In adults this is normally about 120/80. The blood pressure in children depends on age, but younger children generally have lower blood pressure, and it gradually goes up until it reaches adult levels in the early to mid teens.

Every time your heart contracts to force blood along the arteries, a palpable pulse can be felt in various places of the body. The pulse is present in all arteries, but it is felt most easily in those close to the surface, such as at the wrist (the radial pulse) or in your neck (the carotid pulse).

THE IMMUNE SYSTEM

When tiny organisms such as bacteria or viruses enter your body, you feel the symptoms and signs of infection, such as fever, shivering, sweating, aches and pains and skin rashes. Over the years, as children are exposed to more and more of these organisms during day-to-day activities – such as going to school or playing with other children – they gradually develop immunity to them. Immunity to certain diseases can also be acquired through immunisation (see Chapter 5: Infections).

Your body also has natural defences that help fight off these organisms. For example, bone marrow is involved in the production of the cells that make up blood and some of these, collectively known as white blood cells (WBCs), are involved in fighting infection. These cells recognise the infecting organisms by their surface molecules, which are different for each type of infection, like the fingerprint of a human.

FINDING A PULSE

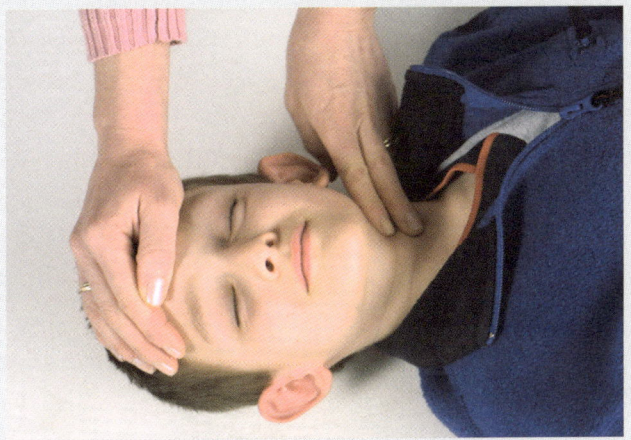

To find the carotid pulse, place two fingers on the 'Adam's apple'. This is felt in the midline of the neck at the front. Slide the tips of your fingers backwards into the groove formed by the neck muscles lying beside the windpipe, as shown above. Apply light pressure and you should feel a pulse.

In very small children, the pulse is often easiest to feel at the side of the upper arm (the brachial pulse) because their necks are short and chubby, making the carotid pulse sometimes difficult to find.

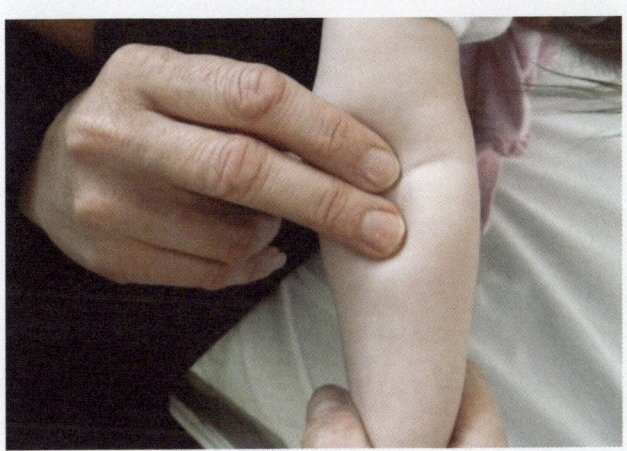

Fighting infections

The first time the body encounters a particular type of infecting organism there is no group of WBCs prepared to fight the intruder, so the body has to make up a new batch specific for that infection.

Some of the WBCs manufacture small pieces of protein known as antibodies, which attach themselves to the infecting organism. They then act as labels to attract the attention of other WBCs that come along and destroy the infecting organism. Because this process depends on the body producing a new batch of WBCs, it usually takes several days of illness before the body has mobilised enough defences to deal with the invading organisms. Once the infection has been defeated some of the specific WBCs die off, as they are not needed in such huge numbers.

There is, however, a small number of each type of WBC stored by the body, as a sort of memory bank for the infection. If your body encounters that same infection again, it can immediately produce the correct WBCs to deal with it. This often occurs without you even realising you have an infection. Exposure to infections goes on all the time – on the bus, at school and work, even at home – as people pass on infectious organisms. This is a necessary process, as the development of immunity protects you from subsequent illness.

Some infections cause such severe disease that you cannot rely on your body's defences alone to fight off the invading organisms. This is why vaccines have been developed to help us become immune to these diseases. These vaccines are often made up of the infecting organisms, but they have been killed and therefore cannot cause infection. Your body can still recognise them, though, and they stimulate your body's immune response.

Although most of the illnesses that cause breathing difficulties are mild and usually resolve themselves without hospital admission or long-term effects, they can become serious. They account for half the visits to GPs and 20 to 30 per cent of hospital admissions for acute childhood illnesses. Respiratory illnesses are also the fifth most common cause of death in children between the ages of one and 14. So it is vital to be able to spot when a child is either severely ill, or has been mildly ill but is getting worse.

2

SIZE MATTERS

How your body works is basically the same from when you are born through to old age, but there are some differences with babies, smaller children, older children and adults.

You need to know about these differences in order to help recognise and treat children who are unwell, and they are especially important when using resuscitation and emergency first aid. In this chapter we explain these important variations, particularly as they relate to breathing and oxygen demand, circulation and body proportions.

Most of the organs in the body, such as the heart and lungs, are smaller in children. However, some – including the liver and spleen – take up relatively more space and therefore they are less protected by ribs and the other parts of the skeleton. This – and the fact that the body wall in children is thinner and more fragile – is important when a child suffers trauma (is injured) because these organs can be more easily damaged than in adults.

AIRWAY

Remember how air passes through your body (see page 22). It starts with an intake of oxygen at your mouth and nose, passes your pharynx, tonsils, larynx and the epiglottis, continues on through your trachea and the two main right and left bronchi, and then down into your lungs, to the alveoli (or the air sacs) at the ends of the smallest airways.

In a child this passageway is much smaller than that of an adult, not only in terms of different body size but also proportionally in relation to the surrounding body parts. For example, a baby's tongue is proportionately much larger inside the mouth than an adult's and their larynx (voice box) is narrower, being funnel-shaped as opposed to an adult's cylindrical-shaped larynx. What this means is that any swelling or obstruction that an adult could deal with without any problem may cause a blockage in the airway of a young child.

Another point of difference is the shape of a baby's head. When compared with older children and adults a baby has a much bigger crown (or occiput), and this makes their head roll forward towards the chest if unsupported when the child is lying flat. The trachea (or windpipe) in adults is held open by solid rings of cartilage but in children it is softer, making it likely to kink if the head is not correctly positioned and is bent forward on the neck. This is of particular relevance in the resuscitation of the infant (see Chapter 24: Basic life support).

BREATHING

The adult chest is a relatively rigid structure because of the ribs and chest wall muscles, which provide support for the lungs. The intercostal muscles (the strong muscles between the ribs) help with movement of the chest when you breathe in (inspiration). In young children, however, the chest wall is still very compliant, or flexible, because the ribs are softer. This reduces the amount of support for their lungs during breathing, making their lungs more liable to collapse.

A child's normal breathing is also more dependent on their diaphragm (the flat muscle separating the abdomen from the chest) than on the intercostal muscles. The extra flexibility of the chest wall is also an important factor when children suffer chest trauma; they are more likely than adults to damage their internal organs (see Chapter 18: Injuries and trauma).

Because the chest wall is flexible, clinical signs of breathing difficulties are more obvious. When a child is ill and struggling to draw breath effectively an 'in-drawing' of their soft tissues can sometimes be seen, especially between the ribs and below the lower edge of the ribcage (this is called 'recession'; see over page). Younger children, especially when exhausted, start to nod their heads as they use the muscles of their neck to help them breathe. Exhaustion due to breathing difficulties is a sign that children are working very hard to breathe – this is a vital sign that you should call for emergency help to prevent them stopping breathing altogether and possibly suffering cardiac arrest.

The respiratory rate, or the amount of breaths per minute, is much higher in children than in adults.

Normal respiratory rates in children

AGE (in years)	RESPIRATORY RATE (breaths per minute)
1 or under	30–40
1 to 2	25–35
2 to 5	25–30
5 to 12	20–25
Over 12	12–20

It is crucial to understand the different breathing rates for the various ages, as an abnormally high or low respiratory rate is an important indicator of the severity of many childhood illnesses (see Chapter 7: Breathing difficulties). To evaluate sick children in an emergency requires you to know their normal breathing rates (see above) so you can recognise an abnormal breathing rate.

The muscles in the abdomen between the ribs (the intercostal muscles) contract when a baby is short of breath. This indrawing of muscles is known as 'intercostal recession' and is a sign of respiratory distress.

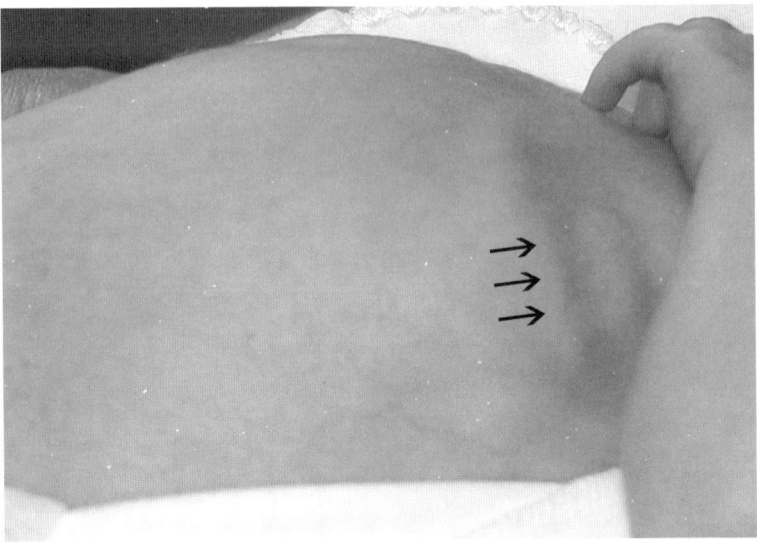

The muscles in the abdomen below the ribs (the subcostal muscles) contract when a baby is short of breath. This is known as 'subcostal recession'.

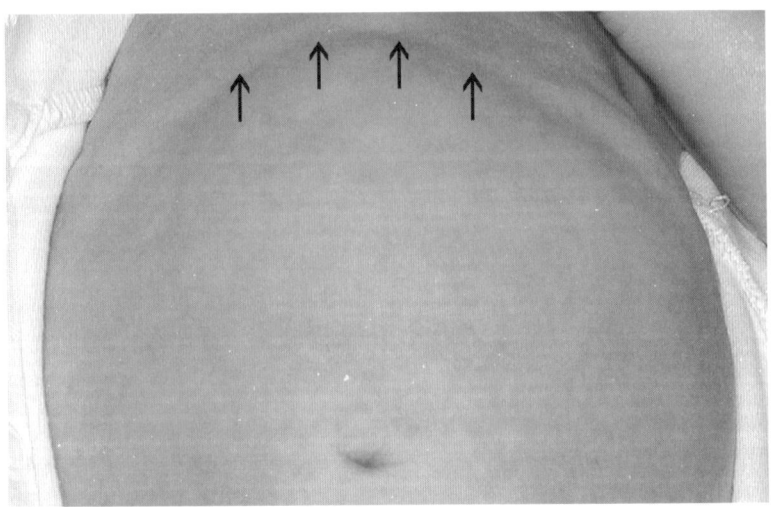

Oxygen demand

Children have a much higher metabolic rate (the rate that the body burns calories and demands oxygen for normal bodily functions) than adults. As an example, small infants can have a metabolic rate approximately twice that of adults, and this naturally decreases as they grow older and larger. During an illness, if there is a problem getting oxygen to the vital organs (heart, brain and kidneys) and tissues, a younger child will become sick a lot faster than an older child or adult would.

When a child is ill, their demand for oxygen may exceed what their body can take in, worsening the symptoms they are experiencing. This may be due to less oxygen getting into the lungs, or to problems created when less oxygen moves from the lungs into the blood. Both of these scenarios may occur in asthma or respiratory infection. Conversely, if a child's metabolic rate increases, they may experience an increased consumption of oxygen in the blood – for instance, during severe infection or in trauma. This may even occur because of an increased breathing rate, when their body is attempting to compensate for another problem.

SOME CAUSES OF VARIATION IN OXYGEN SUPPLY
Decreased oxygen supply
- asthma
- respiratory infection.

Increased oxygen demand
- trauma
- severe infection.

CIRCULATION

The amount of oxygen delivered to the organs and tissues is related to both your heart rate (the number of heartbeats a minute) and the amount of blood pumped from your heart with each heartbeat. In adults, the amount for each heartbeat can be automatically adjusted

Heart rate relative to age

AGE (in years)	HEART RATE (beats per minute)
Under 2	120–160
2 to 5	100–140
5 to 12	80–120
Over 12	60–100

according to demand, but in small children the only way to increase blood flow from the heart is to increase the heart rate. This means that when a child is ill their heart rate increases to compensate for their body's raised demand for oxygen.

The normal heart rate in adults is between 60 to 100 beats per minute, in children aged 5 to 12 years it is 80 to 120 beats per minute, in children aged 2 to 5 years it is 100 to 140 beats per minute, and in children aged one year or younger it is 120 to 160 beats per minute. Knowing this means you will be able to recognise any abnormal heart rate (a high or a low pulse) that may be a clinical sign of illness.

Another important factor is the volume of blood in the body. Taking body weight into consideration, the amount of blood is proportionally higher in children than adults, but the volume of blood is much less in children as their bodies are so much smaller. For each kilogram of body weight an adult has about 70 millilitres of blood, whereas children have 80 millilitres. However, adults have a total of about 5000 millilitres of blood circulating through their bodies, whereas a one-year-old child weighing about 10 kilograms has only 800 millilitres. This has important implications because a child's health can become seriously compromised if they lose relatively small amounts of fluid. This is not only when they bleed but also during illnesses that cause dehydration, such as diarrhoea or vomiting, where deceptively large amounts of fluids may be lost from the bowels.

BODY PROPORTIONS

At birth the head accounts for about a fifth of the body surface area (BSA), whereas in an adult it is about a tenth. Therefore a baby's

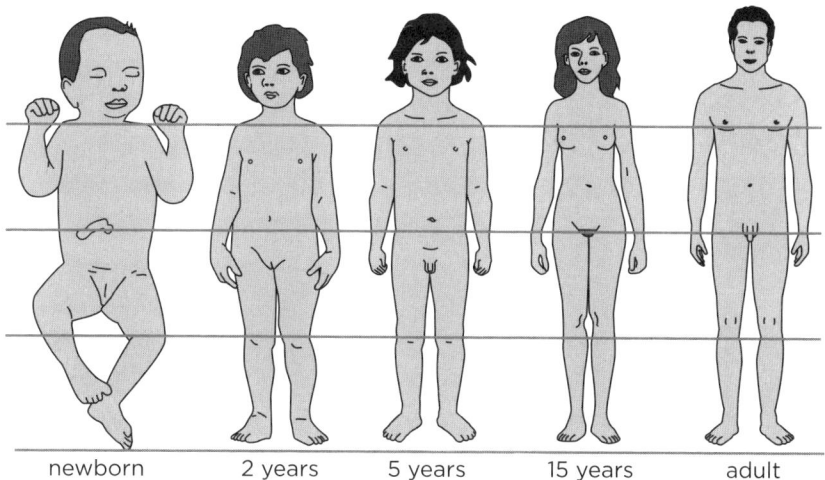

| newborn | 2 years | 5 years | 15 years | adult |

The proportions of the body change with age. In proportion to the rest of their bodies, children have larger heads than adults. And they have a larger body surface compared to volume, which means they can lose heat faster than adults.

head has twice the relative surface area than an adult's. The rest of a child's BSA is also relatively greater than adults. Children obviously weigh much less than adults and this means they have a large BSA-to-volume ratio. So a child has a relatively small amount of valuable body fluid and a large surface area from which to lose it.

Because a large amount of the body's heat is lost from the skin, and because of this proportionately higher body surface area in children, heat loss occurs faster in children than it does in adults. This is a serious problem during childhood illness and this is why it is very important to keep children warm if they are ill or injured.

3

GROWING UP

As children grow, they reach developmental milestones. Apart from the obvious weight and height gains many more subtle changes take place inside your child's body, particularly in the nervous, musculoskeletal, respiratory, cardiovascular, endocrine and immune systems, which are all developing and altering to accommodate the changing functions associated with growth.

From a medical point of view, the changes children go through as they grow are most significant in their immune and neurological systems, followed by age-specific behaviour patterns. It is important to recognise these changes. Doctors rely very heavily on working out any variations from normal appearance and behaviour to determine if a child has a medical problem, and then they use more sensitive tools such as clinical examination and laboratory tests to find out what is causing the problem.

As your child grows their susceptibility to illness and injury also adjusts, as does their body's ability to cope and heal. Birth to

The key divisions of a child's life

STAGE	AGE
Neonate	First 28 days
Waking up	2 to 3 months
The crawler	3 to 18 months
The toddler	18 months to 3 years
The preschooler	3 to 5 years
The schoolchild	5 to 8 years
Prepubescence	8 to 12 years
Puberty	12 years to adulthood

adolescence benchmarks are used by medical professionals to assess any symptoms a child is experiencing and will also be useful for you to help assess your child's health and wellbeing, and to interpret symptoms and signs of illness.

NEONATE: FIRST 28 DAYS

This is probably the most terrifying time for parents. At this age babies don't seem to do much other than sleep, suckle and make pee and poo. In this early period the biggest risk is infection because the immune system is still immature and cannot localise – and therefore control – infection. What this means is that any bacterial infection may be life threatening for a baby this young.

The key to recognising problems early is noticing changes in 'normal' patterns of feeding and behaviour (including sleeping and level of alertness). Even at this very early stage, changes are noticeable. It is important to seek advice at the earliest sign of anything abnormal. More often than not the consultation with a doctor shows that nothing is wrong. However, this should never prevent you seeing a medical practitioner if you have any concerns. If infection is suspected in the newborn, a battery of tests will be performed and broad-spectrum antibiotics promptly prescribed.

There are a number of congenital issues (conditions that the baby is born with) that may become apparent at this time, but rather than attempting to remember all the many different things that could go wrong it is more important to know normal appearance, behaviour and physiology, and thus be able to recognise change. This ability begins with your own experience and knowledge, and that of your family, and continues on to the specialist paediatricians, who also rely on recognition of normal patterns but have great experience of abnormal patterns that can be the pointers for a diagnosis.

WAKING UP: FIRST 3 MONTHS

During this period a baby starts to 'wake up', which means they become more responsive and start to really smile as a response to stimulus rather than make the early baby grimaces. At this age a pattern of behaviour and a schedule for feeding and sleeping fall into place, which may include at least some opportunity for the parents to sleep. A baby's sight also becomes more developed and the baby's muscle tone is increasing, as is the amount of wriggling.

The immune system is still immature but infections are more readily dealt with, and there is now some element of localisation. This means that different disease processes can often be contained within the body system they infect; however, this is not always true and generalised severe illness and sepsis (infection that affects the whole body) are still a problem. Disease at this age is more recognisable by medical practitioners.

Because of your baby's increasing size, lots of wriggling and the fact that you take them out to more places, they are more at risk of being dropped or rolling off flat surfaces. You need to start to be more consistently vigilant when you change nappies, for example, although babies of this age do not roll spontaneously.

THE CRAWLER: 3 TO 18 MONTHS

At this age babies are starting to explore their boundaries and there are many different ways they move along the ground, from crawling to bum shuffling – all of which are probably normal. At some time, from about 8 months through to after 18 months of age, babies will start to pull themselves up to stand and to take their first steps. When this happens it usually has no bearing on their overall development or on disease processes; however, significant delays and any concerns you might have about their ability should always be discussed with your medical practitioner.

The major transition at this age is related to their food – and the increasing variety of available nutrients and proteins when they move on to solids. This can be a seamless process or a nightmare, depending on your luck, but when things go wrong the key is to seek advice from someone you trust. Do not be persuaded to swing too much towards any particular point of view, unless it is based on sound advice. Most importantly, trust your instincts and if you feel something significant is wrong, tell your medical practitioner about your concerns.

Because of the child's extra mobility, there is a very large increase in the risk of trauma and exposure to dangerous situations. By this point a baby's immune system will have developed to a point where it can localise bacterial infections, and illness can be easier to see simply because the baby does a lot more and exhibits an increasing number of typical behaviours, which means change is easy to recognise. Medical practitioners will often do less testing at this age and may adopt a wait-and-see approach if the child looks fine, appears to eat and drink well and is normal when physically examined.

THE TODDLER: 18 MONTHS TO 3 YEARS

This dramatic age is often punctuated by the 'terrible twos' – or 'threes' – and children of this age are predominantly fast moving, attitude filled, lovable monsters with no perception of consequence or danger. This age is characterised by so many bumps to the head that most parents at some stage consider a permanent helmet and various types of body armour. For the most part, toddlers survive this period with a variable collection of scars to the chin and forehead, depending on their nature and their eagerness to explore and take risks.

The key to safety lies in you anticipating and having a high index of suspicion for any circumstances that may be potentially harmful. Keeping them away from major danger – swimming pools, hot things (mostly water and fires) and cars heading the list – means you often can't relax. It is vital to use all available home aids, risk management tools and injury prevention equipment to keep your child from danger, as at this age they will not learn from injury. The best approach is to keep them out of harm's way. (See also Chapter 17: Injury prevention.)

Medically, children at this age have become much more robust, and the typical 'chubby' toddler is fairly indestructible. As always you must be aware of changes in their normal patterns. Providing a brief medical history to a doctor may be very helpful in this age group (as at all ages) as you know your child far better than any examining physician. Your perceptions, observations and concerns are part of any formulation about an illness or on what to do next.

Children in this age group tend be quite gregarious and some will interact with strangers, but others can be very shy. Their immune system is now very developed and a physical examination is usually far more reliable than previously for including and excluding body-system problems. Your treating physician may rely much more heavily on history and examination, with perhaps investigations such as a urine sample to make decisions about treatment and disposition ('where-to-now').

THE PRESCHOOLER: 3 TO 5 YEARS

Your toddler is now much more inquisitive and has the speed and height to get into a lot more things. They do have a seed of awareness of possible consequences, but this is still unreliable and one of your eyes should remain on your child at all times. Household poisons present a great danger at any age, but never more so than at this age – simply keep these products out of the way, on a high shelf or locked up in a secure cupboard. As most child-security locks fail at some point or don't get used every time, go for height first but do be aware that preschoolers creatively use all sorts of things for ladders and love to climb, which in itself may be another source of possible significant trauma around the home.

Children in this age group start to communicate a lot better, and often they can tell you the location of pain and discomfort in their bodies and sometimes clear timelines ('It started to hurt just after breakfast'). They will, however, often be more shy than younger children; 'stranger anxiety' can mean your doctor will ask you to get what information you can from your child, and sometimes it may even be better if they leave the room while you do this.

The preschooler will have developed a strong immune system, which works to localise and contain infection. Therefore, the medical approach to a sick child in this age group is similar to that of an adult. Tests may not need to be done (other than urine tests) and a wait-and-see approach may be the best course of action, assuming the child meets all the safety criteria of eating, drinking, peeing and behaving near normally.

Often at this age children spend substantial amounts of time in childcare and the sharing of childhood viruses begins. Usually there are five to nine episodes per year and the mild fever and snotty nose that characterise this age group may seem continuous at times, but this will pass after a couple of years.

THE SCHOOLCHILD: 5 TO 8 YEARS

A lot of emotional changes happen during this stage of starting school, making friends and developing a vocabulary. It is a time that gives you a lot more insight into your child. It is difficult to protect them because you will not have them in your field of vision all the time, or indeed for much of the time. They ride bikes and skateboards and seem to love speed. Helmets are important – they do save lives – and if you want your children to wear one you must set a good example by wearing one too when you ride a bike. Trauma is the biggest threat due to the age group's risk-taking and adventurous behaviour, and because their immune system is beginning to function at the level of an adult's.

You should discuss the consequences of behaviour regularly with your children as they do have a greater awareness of danger. Unfortunately, this is not 100 per cent reliable so you need to continue to supervise them as much as possible, especially when they are planning their activities. Strong positive reinforcement of good decision-making is much more effective than punishment of bad behaviour, but it is still okay for your child to know you are upset about something they have done that put them in danger.

There is an immense amount of energy in children of their age group and a balanced diet and plenty of physical activity will enhance their development. Some consider computer games, television and DVDs as contemporary blights on an active childhood, and if you set – and stick to – limits on their use early it may help to place these activities in perspective; however, these activities are certainly good on occasion, especially for peace and quiet! (And encourage them to spend some time reading.)

PREPUBESCENCE: 8 TO 12 YEARS

Bicycles, motor vehicles, skateboards, television and peer pressure shape this time of life, and children in this age bracket seem to most parents so much more mature than previous generations. The internet and attendant information overload (often not all age appropriate) may promote many risky activities, from minor behavioural issues to significant and life-threatening endeavours. Early sexual experimentation and the use of social drugs, which were previously more closely related to the puberty years, could become issues. You may need to discuss these issues with your child in a safe and supportive context.

Depression and eating disorders can also occur at this age, possibilities that should be taken seriously. Any suspicion that there may be such a problem needs to be dealt with by an expert. (See also Chapter 16: Mental health problems.)

Medically, this group is approaching adulthood and this is the way health professionals deal with them and assess the possibility of illness. The key element in successful health care is good communication with your medical practitioner, both through you and directly with the child.

PUBERTY AND BEYOND: 12 YEARS TO ADULTHOOD

Bad attitudes and silence have to be dealt with by most parents of teenagers, and fears and concerns about social problems and drug use are common (and they are already looking at your car!). Behaviour at this age tends to change as quickly as the fashionable cut of jeans, and what suited you and the various generations before those of your child do not fit any more.

Parents are getting older, with an increasing trend to starting families later, and a lot of us may be dealing with teenagers when we are in our 50s or 60s, vainly hoping they may go easy on us. No matter what your circumstances, it is vitally important to keep the lines of communication open with constant and non-judgemental interaction – that will increase your chances of not only knowing when something major is going on but hopefully of knowing it in time. It is dangerous to be dogmatic and to stick to your ideas and ideals, which unfortunately at this stage (and probably only temporarily) may not match those of your teenagers.

Glandular fever is commonly contracted at this age, with the frequent and regular exchange of saliva. Providing your children with a good health education, particularly regarding abstinence, safe sex and contraception, can protect them from sexually transmitted disease and teenage pregnancy. Remain open about this and do what you can to educate your children within any religious and moral boundaries you may have.

PART II

YOUR UNWELL CHILD

You can recognise when your child is sick by looking more closely at the illnesses they may get and the way they could respond to them. Chapter 4 is a very important guide to assessing the symptoms and signs of illness, and how these will alert you to whether your child is becoming unwell and how serious it might be. Subsequent chapters break illness down into the common symptoms – infections, fevers, breathing difficulties, abdominal pain, vomiting and diarrhoea, earaches and hearing problems, sore throats and swollen glands, fits and faints, headaches, eye problems, rashes and skin conditions, and mental health problems – and outline causes and treatment.

The more you are aware of possible complications, the more you will be able to prevent or overcome them. This includes recognising the differences between children and adults, not only physically but also in the way children respond to illness. For example, in dealing with young children, there are often communication problems, not only in that children cannot understand what is happening, but also that they cannot express exactly what is wrong. Fear often plays a prominent role in children's illness, and pain cannot be rationalised in the same way it can in adults.

But first of all it is important to look at what makes children sick, and the signs and symptoms to look for to detect difficulties.

4

How to recognise
a seriously ill child

It is important for you to be able to correctly assess your child's health so you can recognise when they are seriously ill. Before moving on to specific symptoms there are some principles that apply to all ill and injured children, and these will be helpful in your ability to gauge when something is wrong.

It is important to have some knowledge of what is normal for your child as this will enable you to more rapidly detect what is abnormal. You need to understand that children have a remarkable ability to compensate when they are sick and may often appear to be well for a considerable period before deteriorating rapidly. The vast majority of babies are born with a 'perfect' physiology (the processes that control how the body works) and are very efficient at using food and oxygen to produce energy and growth. This means children are able to tolerate 'insults' to their bodies from illnesses and injuries that would cause an adult to quickly become very ill. Examples include infections over the age of two to three years or traumatic injury.

The downside of this is that children compensate for illness and injury for some time without showing changes to their health, but when they run out of the capacity to compensate for the problem they become critically ill extremely quickly. When children actually lose the capacity to compensate, they become much more difficult to treat and therefore it is essential that deterioration is identified as soon as possible. Being able to recognise actual and potential problems at this time is the key to saving a child's life.

Another important point is that children often become critically ill – and even die – due to causes that are eminently treatable. The classic symptoms before cardiac arrest in children are hypoxia (lack of oxygen) and hypovolaemia (lack of body fluids). Both of these may be identified early, and if they are diagnosed and treated a situation where a child needs resuscitation may be avoided.

So children and adults are very different in their capacity towards illness and coping ability. Children:

- respond very differently to adults who may have the same illnesses
- can respond very unpredictably when unwell
- can compensate effectively for a long time
- can deteriorate very rapidly when they are seriously unwell.

WHAT MAKES CHILDREN SICK?

The mechanisms (or causes) of illness in children are very different from those that affect adults, mainly because of the way their anatomy and physiology differs. The common illnesses and chronic conditions that affect adults (such as heart disease, emphysema and cancer) are mostly caused by factors associated with normal ageing and lifestyle choices (such as smoking), which gradually deteriorate health over time and can ultimately cause death – and these have obviously not had time to develop in children.

Heart attacks in adults are usually due to atheroma ('furring' or hardening of the arteries), a disease that gradually causes blockages of the arteries which supply blood and oxygen to the heart muscle. Smoking, diabetes and high blood pressure increase the risk of this developing. When children experience life-threatening illness and cardiac arrest, it is rarely caused by this sort of process because atheroma takes many years to develop. Cardiac arrest in children usually follows another illness – involving the lungs, a generalised infection or as a result of significant trauma.

So childhood cardiac arrest is not only less common, it is potentially preventable as long as you are alert to the possible dangers of it when the child is experiencing a serious illness. Therefore the idea that 'children are just small adults' is not true when talking about illness and injury.

Illnesses specific to age

Different types of illnesses in children can generally be grouped according to age. For instance, children of different ages can display similar symptoms that are caused by different diseases, so it is important to have an understanding of which conditions are the most likely in a specific age group. An example of this is the child with a wheeze.

Age-specific causes of wheezing

AGE	CAUSE OF WHEEZE
Under 1 year	Bronchiolitis Inhaled foreign body Allergy/anaphylaxis
Over 1 year	Asthma Allergy/anaphylaxis

Whereas death is often anticipated at the end stage of a chronic disease in adults, especially in the elderly population, very few childhood deaths are 'expected' (with the obvious exception being childhood cancers). Awareness of potential childhood illnesses and recognising the signs when a child's health deteriorates will help in the prevention of events that may cause death, such as heart attacks.

In infants – those under 12 months – the second highest number of deaths are due to cot death. This may be caused by previously unrecognised lung or metabolic problems, or possibly by Sudden Infant Death Syndrome (SIDS), for which typically no cause is found. There are several well-recognised risk factors for cot death, including parental cigarette smoking and the baby sleeping, face-down, on the stomach. Avoiding these risks has reduced the incidence of the condition.

Problems arising from abnormal development in the womb and overwhelming infection are the other main causes of death in this age group. Young children have an immature immune system that makes them less able to defend themselves against infective organisms.

In the slightly older age group, between one and five years old, accidents cause the majority of deaths. This is because at around the age of one year, children start to become mobile but do not yet understand how dangerous the world around them may be. As a child starts to walk, stairs, cars and corners of furniture become new dangers (see Chapter 17: Injury prevention). The other main cause of mortality in this age group is infection, again because the immune system is still relatively immature and is not able to fight off the more severe infections.

In five to 12 year olds, as the child becomes increasingly mobile and gets more adventurous, accidents become by far the biggest danger. Infections pose a proportionately smaller danger than for younger children, as the immune system in this older age bracket matures and is able to fend off more infections.

With children over 12, the pattern of illness becomes similar to young adults, with the predominant cause of death being trauma. The majority of trauma patients are the victims of road traffic accidents, either as pedestrians, cyclists or drivers or passengers in motor vehicles.

TAKING A HISTORY

Monitoring your child and noting down the onset of illness, its severity, its progression and any trends are important indicators of whether they are getting worse, getting better or staying the same. Abnormal signs and the trends you have spotted will also help you decide whether to seek help by seeing your doctor, going to an emergency department or calling the emergency number.

Certain factors in the history of the illness or injury really help with the diagnosis. The normal range of breathing rate, pulse rate and blood pressure are different according to how old a child is (see Chapter 2: Size matters). Although this might make determining the level of illness in a child a little more challenging, any changes noted over time are invaluable in helping to put together an informed picture of their health. An essential part of determining whether any condition affecting a child is serious is the history of the problem.

The 'history' is the story describing the problem, from its first signs. There are some parts of the history that are essential in working out how serious a problem is. Being able to assess and gauge the level of illness or injury of a child by taking a history also means being able to adequately and effectively communicate this to healthcare professionals to enable them to fully appreciate your concerns. It is an essential part of the process. A concise description of how the child's problem has developed with time lines will not only give important information to health professionals, it should also make them realise that you have concerns that need to be taken seriously.

There are certain key points that determine whether a problem is urgent or not:

- onset
- severity
- progression
- response and activity.

Onset
Some medical problems begin suddenly, some may have a gradual onset.

Sudden onset often means that the beginning of a problem is clear; occasionally a child or a carer may even remember the exact time that it started.

Medical problems that have a gradual onset are those where the beginning may not be precisely remembered or able to be pinpointed, but an awareness of its existence gradually became clear. Sudden onset problems are often caused by a break in a bone or a blockage in an organ, whereas gradual onset problems may be caused by a process that gradually builds up, such as infection or inflammation.

With some complaints a sudden onset of symptoms – especially headache, difficulty breathing or swallowing, and pains in the chest or abdomen – suggests that there is a serious problem. Most causes of sudden pain are more common in adults than children, but when they occur in children they should be taken seriously.

Severity

If a child complains that a problem is severe, or if it appears severe to you, it is likely this reflects its true severity. Medical personnel are aware that often a parent, carer and teacher are the people most familiar with the child when they are normal, and so they are the most sensitive judges of when a problem is severe.

As a rough rule of thumb, when the problem drives everything else out of the child's mind, and they cannot concentrate on normal behaviours and activities because of the problem, it is severe or serious.

A good example is abdominal pain. All children suffer abdominal pain of some description at one time or another, but they can almost always pay attention to other things going on, even if it is to react to their parents, respond relatively normally, talk, laugh, pay attention and so on. When the pain is severe, it occupies their mind to the exclusion of all of these things and makes normal interaction impossible.

Progression

A problem may have a sudden or a gradual onset, but a very important aspect of its description is how it progresses after its onset.

Non-serious problems have symptoms that tend to undulate, or come and go, as the body makes attempts to deal with the causes of the disease. More serious problems are defined by becoming constant, or growing steadily worse over time, whether they are a sudden or gradual onset.

When medications are given, such as paracetamol or ibuprofen, symptoms are often relieved temporarily and it is easy to think that this has solved the problem. Certainly treatments such as these are essential for comfort; however, bear in mind that the progression of the disease is not altered – it is only masked for periods, and must be monitored.

Response and activity

A good way to judge whether an illness is severe or not is whether a child is able to respond appropriately to stimuli, especially in reaction to parents and siblings. Children who can play normally, are alert, talkative and interested in their surroundings are seldom seriously ill, at least at this point. However, it is also important to realise that this may change and that it is vital to keep reassessing the child's interaction and responsiveness at regular intervals, and to be aware of any reduction in alertness.

THE IMPORTANCE OF TRENDS

When taking a history you need to take notice of trends or patterns – it may be changes in the wheeziness from asthma, a rash from an allergic reaction, breathing rate from bronchiolitis or croup, fever from any infection, or level of consciousness in a head injury. But keep in mind that children have different rates of breathing, pulse and blood pressure, depending on their size (see Chapter 2: Size matters). Young children, particularly babies and infants, have much higher breathing and pulse rates than older children, for instance. So it is important to have some sense of what their normal range is as you need to be able to identify when these measurements become abnormal.

Breathing rates and pulse rates should always be measured more than once, because even in normal children and adults they can be quite different from one moment to the next. The average of all measurements taken should be within the normal ranges. But because a child's ability to compensate for injury, disease and illness is so good, measured variables such as breathing rate may actually never go into the abnormal range.

Normal physiology also includes level of consciousness, or being awake and alert at the right times. Younger children need more sleep than adults, with babies, infants and toddlers usually sleeping in the daytime as well as at night, but even teenagers need at least 8 to 10 hours of sleep a night to maintain normal growth and function. If a child is ill, they may be miserable and may want to sleep more, but they still should have a normal level of consciousness. This is where the AVPU scheme comes into play. The letters stands for:

- **A**lert
- responds to **V**oice
- responds to **P**ain
- **U**nresponsive.

This is a way for health professionals to assess the patient's level of consciousness: each level describes an incremental decrease in conscious level. Children should always be in the Alert category – if asleep they should be in the Voice category. Anything outside this is abnormal.

A trend, by definition, is at least *three* measurements of something, so it is important to repeatedly measure or estimate whatever you are assessing. Although children have highly effective systems that can compensate for all sorts of illnesses and injuries, they do lose their ability to compensate if they deteriorate. The period leading up to this loss of compensation, and even the initial stages of abnormality, can be spotted and dealt with effectively if you are observing and taking notice of trends.

QUICK REFERENCE
How to take a pulse, see page 31.
Measuring breathing, see page 97.
See page 102 for more information on AVPU.

HOW AND WHEN TO REACT

It is absolutely normal and expected for parents to be on high alert for any potential harm that may come to their children, and this alertness extends to anyone who cares for a child. We all know that children are more vulnerable than adults, and that for various reasons they – or their bodies – do not have the same abilities to defend themselves against infection, illness and injury. It is even more important then to be sensitive to the signs of severe illness and the signs that reveal worsening illness while still being accurate in your assessment and description of the problem. This will really help you to know when to do something about the illness, and how to communicate this to healthcare professionals. (For a general outline of how to do this, see Chapter 25: Handing over to the professionals.)

Doctors and nurses in emergency departments and paramedics are taught a process of triage, which is a French word for 'to sort'. It means they systematically assess the medical history and examine a sick child. By doing so they estimate the level of illness. Doctors and nurses who do not work in emergency departments are not generally taught to work in this manner, and therefore they may not be as sensitive to the important aspects of a history of illness or to the important changes that occur and may be seen in the examination of a sick or injured child.

A very good way to transmit this information is to keep your own notes to help you describe the problems. Even though, when your child is sick or injured, it may seem impossible to think about writing things down, it may prove to be one of the most important things you can do for them.

Handover notes

A description of what you or others have done to intervene and treat the child, if anything, provides health professionals a lot of insight into how unwell the child is. This may range from administering paracetamol through to basic life support. This summary of the child's medical history, including medications, allergies and operations, is very useful. See the sample handover sheet, with simple headings to guide you in how to compile this information, on the following page.

When to go to your GP or hospital or call for help

Uppermost in your mind when dealing with a sick child should be this question:

• Are you very worried about them?

SAMPLE HANDOVER SHEET

HISTORY	
Onset	Sudden/gradual? Time: _____ Date: _____
Progression	Increased? Decreased? Constant? Intermittent?
Severity	At beginning? Now? Trend?
Response and activity	Normally reacting to stimuli? Alert? Smiling? Playing? Moving? Feeding? Drinking? Trend?
SIGNS	
Airway	Normal? Swelling around mouth? Drooling? Noisy? Trend?
Breathing	Fast/slow? Recession? Tiredness/ exhaustion? Trend?
Circulation	Colour: pale/flushed/rash? Sweaty? Pulse rate? Trend?
Dysfunction	Level of consciousness (AVPU)? Changes/trends?
Exposure	Rash? Injury seen: bruising, bleeding, cuts and grazes, deformity (bones)?
Medications given	Paracetamol? Ibuprofen? Other? Effect?
KNOWN MEDICAL HISTORY	
Previous illnesses	Previous and current treatments?
Medications	Previous and current?
Operations	What? When? Why?
Allergies	What to? What happens? Any treatment (such as an adrenaline injection for severe allergies)?

A side effect of teaching parents and other carers how to identify the history and signs of serious illness and injury may be that they are less concerned if their children appear well. You may have taken a careful history and identified trends, but these findings should always be superseded by anything that unsettles you even if you can't put your finger on what it is.

If you are very concerned about them for any reason, even if they have none of the worrying history or signs we have described, that is enough of a reason to either take them to your doctor, a hospital or call 000 (111 in New Zealand). No doctor, nurse or paramedic who is well trained in paediatric emergencies would ever criticise you for behaving in this way.

Deciding to go to an emergency department rather than call the emergency number depends on whether you believe there is a need for immediate treatment – it is likely an ambulance could get to you and provide immediate resuscitation with treatments such as adrenaline before you could reach the hospital.

If you go to the hospital under your own steam you will be triaged. That means a health professional (usually a nurse) will decide whether you need immediate treatment or can wait for treatment. You will be triaged as urgent if your child's condition is more severe than you recognised and then will be treated accordingly; if your child is not so unwell, you may have to wait to be seen by the doctor.

THE DIFFERENCE BETWEEN SYMPTOMS AND SIGNS

The symptoms are the components of information you gather from the patient or their story about the disease; the signs are what you see or feel. So, for example, a symptom is pain but a sign is the tenderness when you feel the abdomen.

The three tables on the following pages describe how you need to react, and who to see or call in certain circumstances.

Remember, if you are very worried about a child, this is reason enough to seek medical help.

When to see your general practitioner

Breathing problem not getting any better after 24 hours

Breathing problem with a cough or fever

A fever associated with a sore throat, sore ears or a cough

Sore throat, sore ears or swollen glands for more than 2 days

---

Any pain for more than 2 days despite receiving adequate paracetamol or ibuprofen

---

Vomiting or diarrhoea for more than 24 hours

Abdominal pain and not eating or drinking

Headache but no rash and a normal level of consciousness

If you are concerned that you may not be able to spot any worrying symptoms in your child

---

If you are worried about your child and would like expert advice

---

When to go to the emergency department

Breathing problems with the child breathing quickly or finding it difficult to breathe normally

---

Breathing problems with a high fever

Abdominal pain that moves from one part of the tummy to another

---

Vomiting that is increasing in frequency

Diarrhoea for 3 days or more

A rash and a fever but otherwise well

A fit or a faint if you are not sure what has caused it

Fainting during exercise or exertion

A high fever (greater than 39°C)

A severe headache

If you are VERY worried about your child and would like them to be checked out

---

When to call the emergency number – 000 in Australia, 111 in New Zealand

---

If your child is unresponsive and not breathing – START BASIC LIFE SUPPORT

Breathing problems and the child is becoming quiet or exhausted

---

Breathing problems and blue lips

Breathing problems that are rapidly becoming worse

Severe abdominal pain that you cannot control

A rash associated with a fit or a decrease in the level of consciousness

---

A high fever associated with a fit or a decrease in the level of consciousness

---

Not fully regaining full consciousness after a fit or a faint

---

A pink raised rash and difficulty breathing after a bite or a sting

---

If you are EXTREMELY worried about your child and think they need medical attention immediately

---

5

INFECTIONS

Infection is one of the most important and common causes of disease and death in childhood. Every child will suffer from a multitude of infections, ranging from the common cold to infected cuts and grazes, and from tonsillitis to common childhood rashes such as measles or chicken pox. Most of these are unlikely to cause significant harm, but there are certain signs and symptoms that give early warning of serious illness.

WHAT IS AN INFECTION?
Infections are caused by tiny organisms, such as bacteria or viruses, that enter the body. The immune system is the body's weapon to resist these infections (see Chapter 1: How the body works). Children build immunity gradually during their early years as they are exposed to more and more of these organisms from their family and friends, and when they play with other children and go to day-care, preschool and school. Their body remembers the organism it was affected by

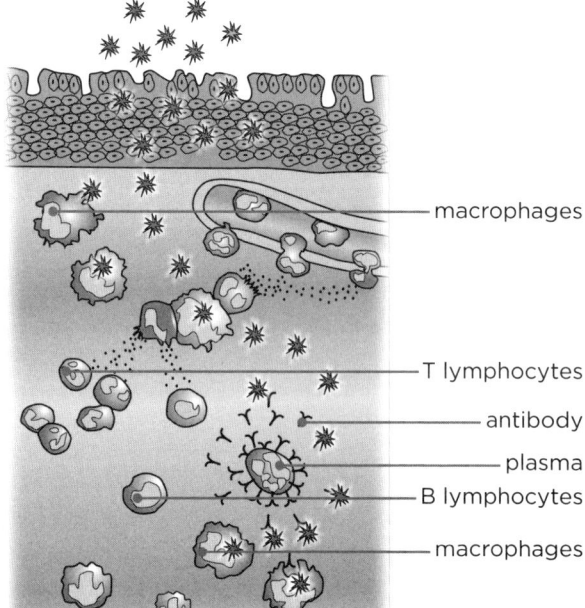

macrophages

T lymphocytes

antibody

plasma

B lymphocytes

macrophages

Infecting organisms are targeted by T and B lymphocytes (white blood cells) and macrophages (specialised cells in the tissues).

and mounts a defence initially, then remembers the organism and responds (more effectively) when it reappears. This process minimises the harm done to the body by getting rid of the invaders. It is the body's natural defence to help fight off these organisms.

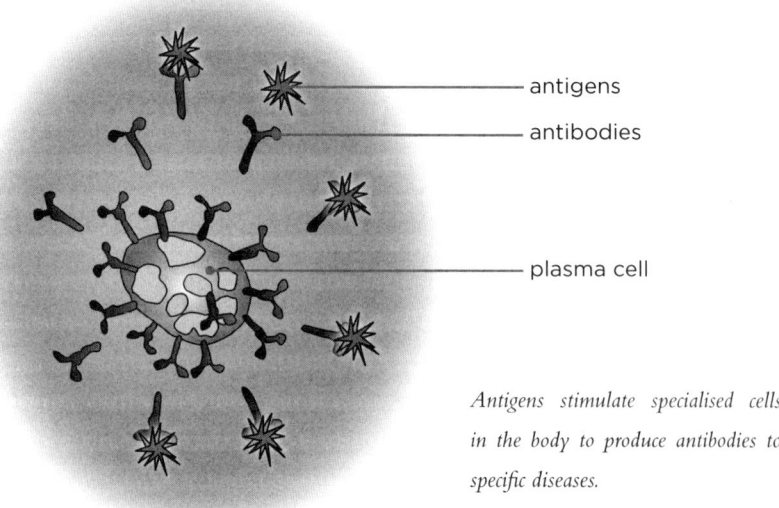

antigens

antibodies

plasma cell

Antigens stimulate specialised cells in the body to produce antibodies to specific diseases.

Symptoms and signs of infection

Usually symptoms are specific to the area of infection; for example, you cough when you have a chest infection and have pain and redness on an area of infected skin. Children, however, may exhibit more general symptoms of infection and sometimes it may not be obvious that something is wrong. Especially in infants, the signs of infection may be subtle and may show up as poor feeding, general lethargy or a decrease in level of responsiveness. A 'floppy baby' should always be assumed to be a sick baby needing medical attention immediately.

The general symptoms of infection are:

- fever
- shivering
- sweating
- aches and pains
- cough
- skin rashes.

HOW INFECTIONS OCCUR

Infection gets into the body by three main routes:

- by breathing in infected droplets from coughs or sneezes
- taken in by mouth in food or drink or from the child's hand after contact with another infected person
- through the skin via breaks in the surface (as in cuts or grazes)
- by contact with infected surfaces.

Infection through breathing in

Although infectious diseases can affect any organ system, the most common route the harmful organisms take to enter the body is via the lungs.

As a person coughs or sneezes, thousands of tiny droplets of saliva are expelled at over 1100 kilometres per hour. If you inhale these droplets, which contain infectious organisms, they get into your body. Examples of infections that are spread in this way are the common cold, influenza, measles and chicken pox. You can see how large

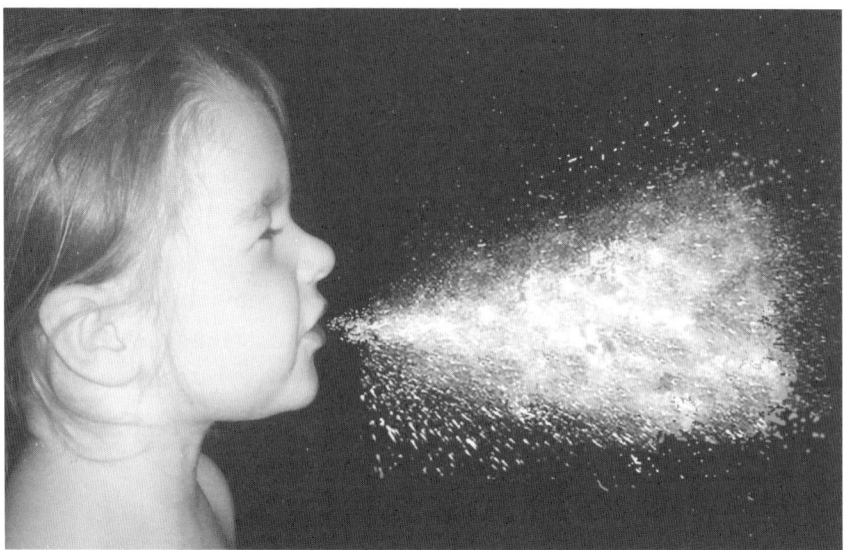

When you sneeze, droplets are expelled at over 1100 kilometres per hour. This is one of the commonest ways that infections are spread.

populations become infected this way, as each infected person may inadvertently spread the disease to many others. In 1666, the Black Death was dispersed in this way.

Oral infections

Most episodes of gastroenteritis (or food poisoning) occur because harmful organisms (or toxins from organisms) have entered the body in food or water, or from the child's hands after contact with contaminated matter such as faeces or with other sick kids. This is often because of poor hygiene by those who prepared or transported the food, but it may also come from other sources. It is difficult to guard against this type of infection, but a great reduction in the infection rates may be achieved by paying attention to simple measures such as adequate hand washing before and after preparing food.

Food standards in our shops and supermarkets are usually extremely high, but washing fruit and vegetables and thorough cooking of meats are always recommended to avoid contamination. In third world countries the spread of disease via the water supply is much more common. Outbreaks of cholera can affect large numbers of people where there is poor sanitation and a contaminated water supply.

Skin infections

The skin forms a continuous layer around the body. In normal circumstances all humans have organisms that live on the skin, causing no harm at all. If the skin is broken (for example, by a cut or graze), these normally harmless organisms may cause infection. You would be familiar with a skin infection as a hot, red, painful swelling, often with a collection of pus under the skin.

BEWARE OBJECTS THAT MAY SPREAD INFECTION

Many inanimate objects may carry disease-causing organisms or germs which then spread infections. You may hear these referred to as fomites. Infection can then be transmitted via droplet, mouth or broken skin. Diseases such as the common cold, conjunctivitis, cold sores, Escherischia coli (E. coli) infections, meningitis, rotavirus and croup can all be transmitted in this way.

The objects that commonly transmit disease are things such as toothbrushes, taps and sinks, and toys. Toys in waiting rooms, day-care centres or kindergartens may have recently been handled by children with contagious organisms, and the habit of young children putting everything in their mouth adds to the risk of transmission. Other common examples at home are tissues, toilets, nappies and cutlery as well as any object that comes into contact with uncooked foods (such as cutting boards).

Organisms may live on these objects for minutes, hours or even days. The best way deal with these risks is to recognise them as opportunities to prevent illness – teach children frequent, effective hand-washing and regularly clean and disinfect objects that come into contact with uncooked food or toileting activities.

Some infections may come from other sources, such as earth or faeces. A particularly severe infection can be caused by tetanus, which is contracted in this way, but vaccination against tetanus reduces this risk considerably. Some illnesses, such as conjunctivitis or bronchiolitis, may be caused by contact transmission and occur when children touch another person with a particular disease or a person or object that has been in contact with someone with the disease.

CHILDHOOD INFECTIONS

Infections can be common, such as coughs and colds, and they can infect various organs in the body. Infection in the gastrointestinal tract can cause vomiting and diarrhoea (see Chapter 9: Vomiting and diarrhoea). Infections in the chest and lungs can cause respiratory problems (see Chapter 7: Breathing difficulties). Infections can also occur in the ears, nose and throat and, rarely, in the brain and spinal cord.

Coughs

Coughs are very common in children. Most children will get five to ten bouts of coughs a year. By far the most common cause of a cough is an upper respiratory tract infection (see 'The common cold' opposite and Chapter 7: Breathing difficulties). These infections are usually caused by a virus, which means that antibiotics have no role in their treatment (they are effective against bacteria only). Some children can cough for up to two weeks following a viral infection. Occasionally coughs may be due to a more serious cause, such as a bacterial infection (for example, pneumonia or tonsillitis), croup or bronchiolitis (see Chapter 7: Breathing difficulties). A persistent night-time cough could be due to asthma.

TREATMENT

If your child is well apart from having a cough, then there is no specific treatment needed. If you are concerned about your child or the duration of their cough, then you should see your local doctor. Be mindful that smoking cigarettes near children can make their cough worse – this should always be avoided.

The common cold

The most prevalent upper respiratory tract infection is the common cold, which can cause a high temperature, sneezing and a runny or blocked nose. Half of all children with runny noses develop a sore throat, and almost half experience a cough. Colds are caused by viruses and are usually caught by hand-to-hand contact, with the infective organisms subsequently reaching the nostrils or eyes via the hands rather than through droplets released by someone's coughing.

TREATMENT

Colds generally require little or no treatment, although the symptoms can be alleviated with medications such as paracetamol or ibuprofen, which are both used to reduce high temperatures. In some instances a simple bulb suction device can be used to clear the nose of secretions and allow for more comfortable breathing. As for coughs, treating the common cold with antibiotics has little effect because the cold is caused by a virus.

Ear infections

Infections of the middle ear (the part of the ear behind the eardrum) are extremely common in childhood, with 20 per cent of children under four years of age being affected at least once a year. These infections are often related to a viral cold-like illness affecting the upper respiratory passages (see page 86), and as there is a link between the back of the throat and the middle ear, infection can travel directly between these two areas. Pus may accumulate in the middle ear space and the eardrum can become tense and swollen.

Recurrent ear infections may lead to glue ear. This is a chronic (long-term) condition in which there is secretion of thick fluid into the middle ear. Glue ear is the most common cause of hearing loss in children and it may interfere with speech development and cause learning difficulties. (See Chapter 14: Earaches and hearing problems.)

TREATMENT

Like the majority of common cold infections it is likely that the cause will be viral rather than bacterial, so the role of antibiotics is uncertain. There is good evidence that antibiotics are not required for this condition unless it has lasted for more than 48 to 72 hours and the child is very unwell. For children with very painful ear infections, local anaesthetic drops can sometimes help to reduce the pain (but this is not a common practice) – seek advice from your local doctor. If the problem persists due to a collection of pus behind the eardrum, it may need to be drained (not during the acute infection but afterwards) by a surgeon placing a small plastic tube through the eardrum, called a grommet.

Throat infections and tonsillitis

Infections of the throat are also common in children. The tonsils in the throat are localised areas of lymphoid tissue. They are part of the immune system responsible for filtering infection from surrounding areas. When there is infection present the tonsils become intensely inflamed, swollen and painful, resulting in tonsillitis.

In tonsillitis, fever may occur and the child may complain of feeling hot, cold, shivery and sweaty, with muscular aches and pains. There may also be marked generalised illness with headache and abdominal pain (which are more likely to occur with a bacterial infection).

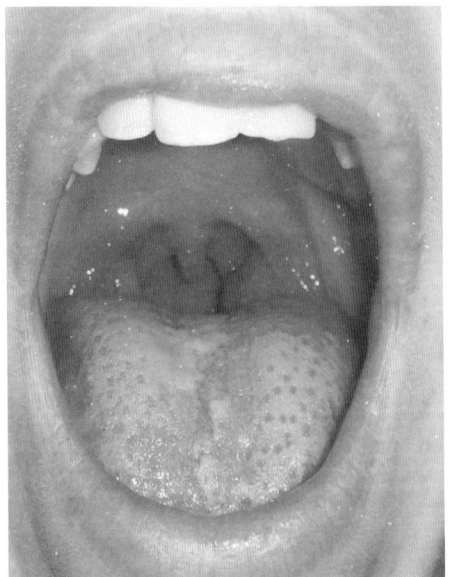

The tonsils lie at the back of the mouth, at the entrance to the pharynx. When infected, they become swollen and red.

TREATMENT

It is not usually possible to tell the difference between bacterial and viral tonsillitis, but the majority of episodes of tonsillitis are caused by viral infection so antibiotics are not usually necessary. General treatment should be aimed at relieving the symptoms with painkillers such as paracetamol or ibuprofen. Aspirin should not be used in children under 12 (as it can lead to damage of the liver and brain). Some doctors feel that penicillin is warranted for a severe infection.

If your child shows any evidence of:

- breathing difficulties, call the emergency number – 000 in Australia, 111 in New Zealand
- not being able to swallow food and drink, especially when there are any signs of dehydration, take them to the nearest emergency department.

Remember, children lose fluids easily, and they often do not have to lose much for this to be a problem.

Infections of the brain and spinal cord

Infection of the lining around the brain and spinal cord – the meninges – leads to a disease known as meningitis. Meningitis may be caused by a variety of organisms, but bacterial meningitis is the most severe and the one discussed here.

Another infection which may affect the brain itself rather than the linings is called encephalitis. Encephalitis is often part of meningo-encephalitis (an infection of both the brain and the tissues surrounding it) and the clinical picture develops along the same lines as meningitis. An abscess can also occur in the brain as in any other part of the body (wherever it is located, an abscess is a localised collection of pus). This condition can affect a child in similar ways to meningitis and for that reason it is not discussed separately. Viral meningitis usually begins in the same way as bacterial meningitis but often progresses less rapidly and the symptoms are vaguer. The distinction between viral and bacterial meningitis is usually only made after a lumbar puncture test of the fluid surrounding the spinal cord and brain.

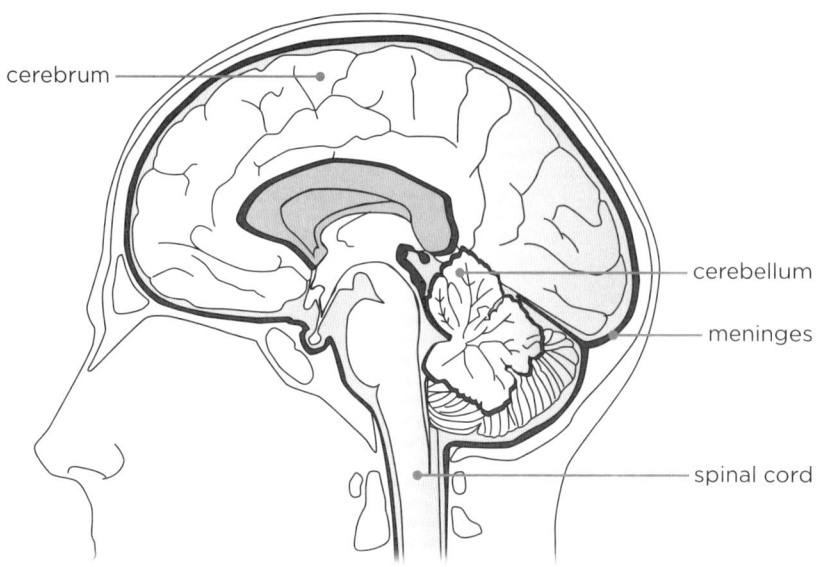

cerebrum

cerebellum

meninges

spinal cord

The meninges is a system of membranes that line and protect the brain and the spinal cord. When infected — usually by viruses or bacteria — it becomes inflamed and causes a number of non-specific symptoms, which often include a rash.

Bacterial meningitis mainly affects children, with over 80 per cent of all patients in Australia being under 16 years of age. As with all children's diseases, awareness and early recognition are the keys to a good outcome. The early symptoms of bacterial meningitis are unfortunately non-specific, especially in infants; for example, fever, poor feeding, vomiting, irritability and drowsiness. Older children complain of headache, symptoms of fever such as shivering, sweating and muscle aches, neck stiffness and an aversion to light (photophobia). A classic sign of meningitis infection is a rash, which most parents will be aware of. This rash is specific in appearance, being red to purple in colour (like a bruise), in small patches the size of a pinhead or slightly larger, and it does not turn white when pressed (for example, when a glass is pressed to the skin).

An infant may go 'floppy' when infected — remember, a floppy baby is a very ill baby — and an older child may be drowsy and less

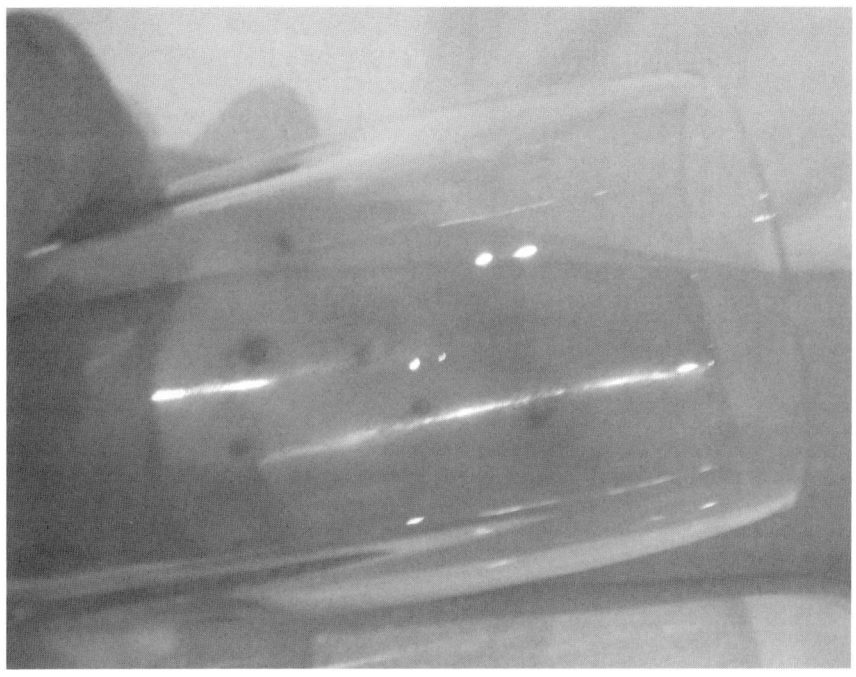

The typical rash associated with meningococcal disease does not fade or blanch when pressed with a glass. It is red to purple, and occurs in numerous small patches the size of a pinhead. A rash is not always present, however.

responsive than usual. Sometimes the child may have a fit (seizure) and become unconscious, and all their limbs start to shake (see Chapter 10: Faints and fits). If meningitis is suspected, your child should be taken to the nearest emergency department. If your child has only mild symptoms – which, however, are enough to make you concerned (for example, has a moderate headache and fever) – you can take them yourself. If they are unstable or very unwell (have a decreased level of consciousness or are very drowsy), call an emergency ambulance – 000 in Australia, 111 in New Zealand.

In certain circumstances, such as you are close to a major hospital with an emergency department or in a rural area with a short travelling time to the local hospital, you may be better off taking the child straight to the emergency department even if they are very unwell.

But the best choice in all circumstances if you are very concerned and your child is very sick is to call 000 (or 111 in New Zealand).

TREATMENT

The treatment of these infections of the brain involves high doses of intravenous antibiotics, aimed at reducing the severity of the illness.

GENERAL INFECTION TREATMENT

The vast majority of infections cause a short period of illness. The body's defences can fight off the infection, resulting in immunity to the same infection in the future. Symptoms that suggest a fever are hot and cold sweats, shivering attacks and generalised muscle aches and pains (see Chapter 6: Fevers).

TREATMENT

In these cases, no treatment is necessary other than to control the symptoms. Paracetamol or ibuprofen should be used to reduce a high temperature and this will also give a degree of pain relief if there is any discomfort (see Chapter 6: Fevers).

Good fluid intake is an important aspect of the treatment of any childhood infection, as children are particularly vulnerable to fluid loss. This is because they have a large surface area compared with a relatively small body fluid volume. Therefore they do not have much fluid to lose, but a lot of skin surface to lose it from. In infective illnesses there may be increased fluid loss from the lungs (through moist air being exhaled), the skin (through sweat) and the gastrointestinal tract (through diarrhoea and vomiting), so the risk of fluid loss is multiplied.

Antibiotics are not necessary in the majority of these illnesses because viruses cause the majority of childhood infections and do not respond to antibiotic treatment. In fact antibiotics have some side effects – for example, they can cause diarrhoea, allergy and rashes – which may be worse than the initial illness itself. Widespread overuse of antibiotics also leads to bacteria becoming resistant to some antibiotics and more difficult to treat (which has led to the development of potent drug-resistant bugs).

IMMUNISATION AS PREVENTATIVE TREATMENT

Immunity is acquired through immunisation programs, preventing the illness from occurring in the first place. Vaccines have been developed for a number of diseases that can cause severe reactions in children.

Recommended Australian immunisation schedule

AGE	VACCINE
Birth	Hepatitis B (hepB)
2 months AND 4 months AND 6 months	Hepatitis B (hepB) Diphtheria, tetanus, pertussis (DTPa) Haemophilus influenza type B (Hib) Polio (oral) Pneumococcus (7vPCV) Rotavirus
12 months	Hepatitis B (hepB) Haemophilus influenza type B (Hib) Measles, mumps, rubella (MMR) Meningococcal C
12 to 24 months	Hepatitis A (Aboriginal and Torres Strait Islanders in high-risk areas)
18 months	Varicella (VZV)
18 to 24 months	Pneumococcus polysaccharide (23vPPV) Hepatitis A (both for Aboriginal and Torres Strait Islanders in high-risk areas)
4 years	Diphtheria, tetanus, pertussis (DTPa) Measles, mumps, rubella (MMR) Polio (oral)
10 to 13 years	Hepatitis B (hepB) Varicella (VZV)
12 to 13 years	Human papilloma virus (HPV)
15 to 17 years	Diphtheria, Tetanus, Pertussis (DTPa)

Immunisation programs have greatly reduced diseases that threaten the lives of children throughout the world and their importance cannot be overemphasised. Smallpox has been all but eradicated by the most comprehensive vaccination program in the world. Diphtheria and pertussis (whooping cough) have declined as threats because of vaccines, and vaccinations have made the current generation of doctors in the western world unlikely to ever see a case of tetanus.

Other vaccinations, though, have failed to eradicate a disease, often because of the particularly resilient nature of the organisms. Tuberculosis is once again on the increase due to many factors, one of which is the decline in the rates of the BCG vaccination, which was phased out in Australia and New Zealand several decades ago.

Parents are often concerned about adverse effects of vaccines. Any possible side effects must be seen in the light of three things:

- how often side effects actually occur and, if they do, how serious they are
- how likely children are to catch the disease if they are not immunised
- the possible consequences of not having the vaccine.

The likelihood of getting the disease if not immunised, and the consequences if that happened, mean that immunisation is by far the safer option. Immunisations that concern parents are the MMR (measles, mumps, rubella) and pertussis (whooping cough) vaccines.

A link between the MMR vaccine and either autism or inflammatory bowel disease has been suggested. At the time of writing, there is no convincing evidence this actually exists. The risk of brain damage linked with the pertussis vaccine is thought to be extremely rare and is, in general, outweighed by the benefits of preventing this potentially fatal disease (especially in very young babies). However, if a child has a history of neurological problems (for example, fits or cerebral palsy), then the vaccine is not recommended.

Further information about the facts behind immunisation can be found at <www.immunise.health.gov.au> and <www.immune. org.nz>.

6

FEVERS

Fever in childhood is very common. It is a part of the body's normal response to an infection (usually by a virus or a bacterium). The important thing with fever in children is to look for the symptoms and signs of a more serious illness rather than just looking at the fever on its own.

WHAT IS A FEVER?

Normal body temperature is 36.5 to 37.5°C. A fever is when the body temperature is higher than 38°C.

As a fever is a normal response by the body to an infection, it occurs when the immune system that fights infection (for example, the white blood cells, plasma cells and antibodies) needs to work more effectively, and it does this at higher temperatures. A fever alone is usually not harmful to your child unless the temperature reaches 42°C or above. A child's temperature will return to normal when the infection that has caused the fever has gone.

HOW FEVERS OCCUR

Most fevers are caused by infection by a virus (the most common) or a bacterium (least common).

Viral infections are responsible for the vast majority of childhood infections. They are associated with milder symptoms, the illnesses are self-limiting (in other words, they get better by themselves) and they do not require treatment. Any viral or bacterial infection can lead to a fever.

The commonest childhood infections are:

- respiratory tract infection (see Chapter 7: Breathing difficulties)
- gastroenteritis (see Chapter 9: Vomiting and diarrhoea)
- ear infections (see Chapter 5: Infections)
- common viral rashes of childhood such as chicken pox, measles, rubella, scarlet fever, mumps (see Chapter 5: Infections)
- appendicitis (see Chapter 8: Abdominal pain)
- urinary tract infection (see Chapter 8: Abdominal pain).

The commonest cause by far for fever in childhood is a viral upper respiratory tract infection (viral URTI). These infections are called by various names, including the common cold, sore throat, tonsillitis and the flu.

A viral URTI can cause worrying symptoms, such as a runny or blocked nose, coughing, ear or sinus pain and fever.

Less common causes of childhood fever are encephalitis and meningitis (see Chapter 10: Faints and fits).

Treating fevers

Most children with a fever will be happy and comfortable and will have only mild symptoms (such as those of a viral URTI).

It is not necessary to treat all fevers; in fact, a fever is actually a good thing most of the time because the cells that the body uses to fight an infection function more efficiently in a slightly raised temperature.

If you do need to make your child more comfortable by reducing their fever, you can try the following methods:

- Dress the child according to their behaviour – if they are shivering, put more clothes on until they stop; if they are sweating, take off their clothes layer by layer.
- Use paracetamol (Panadol), which will reduce your child's temperature. Follow the directions on the bottle – and always make sure you do not give doses more frequently than every four hours, and give no more than four doses in every 24 hours.
- An alternative to paracetamol is ibuprofen (Nurofen) to reduce your child's temperature. Again, the amount given should be as directed on the bottle. There is no evidence that using either paracetamol and ibuprofen together, or alternating doses of paracetamol and ibuprofen, is any more beneficial than using either of them alone.
- Make sure your child has plenty of clear fluids to drink (for example, water or diluted fruit juice). Do not worry if they do not want to eat – giving them lots of fluids is the most important way to help to reduce the fever and to prevent dehydration. Even relatively small children can do without any food for a short while, unless they have diabetes or a similar medical problem.

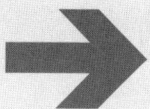

FEVER IN SMALL BABIES
Fever in babies aged three months or younger is managed differently because at this age the immune system is not fully developed and their bodies react to infections differently than those of older children.

It is very important that children of this age who have a fever of over 38°C are seen by a doctor urgently.

Antibiotics do not work to treat a viral infection. Bacterial infections are less common but are usually associated with more significant symptoms than viral infections. Most bacterial infections require treatment with antibiotics.

Unless your child is very unwell and/or feels hot to the touch, it is unnecessary to take their temperature.

HOW TO TAKE A TEMPERATURE

There are different ways to take a child's temperature and many different thermometers to use. Follow the instructions on your thermometer carefully to allow an accurate temperature reading. In general, thermometers that take measurements from under the armpit are more accurate. If you are measuring a temperature from under the tongue make sure the child has not recently had a very hot or very cold drink, as this can lead to a false temperature reading. Thermometers that record from the ear ('tympanic electronic' type thermometers) or the forehead (via adhesive tape) are not as reliable.

- Use a thermometer meant for humans and in functioning order.
- Place the thermometer under the armpit or under the tongue – the most accurate ways to measure temperature.
- Ensure your child has not recently had a hot or cold drink if taking temperature from under the tongue.

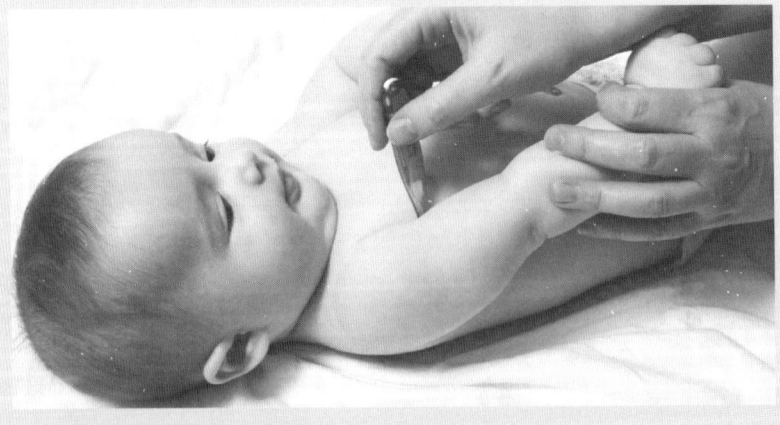

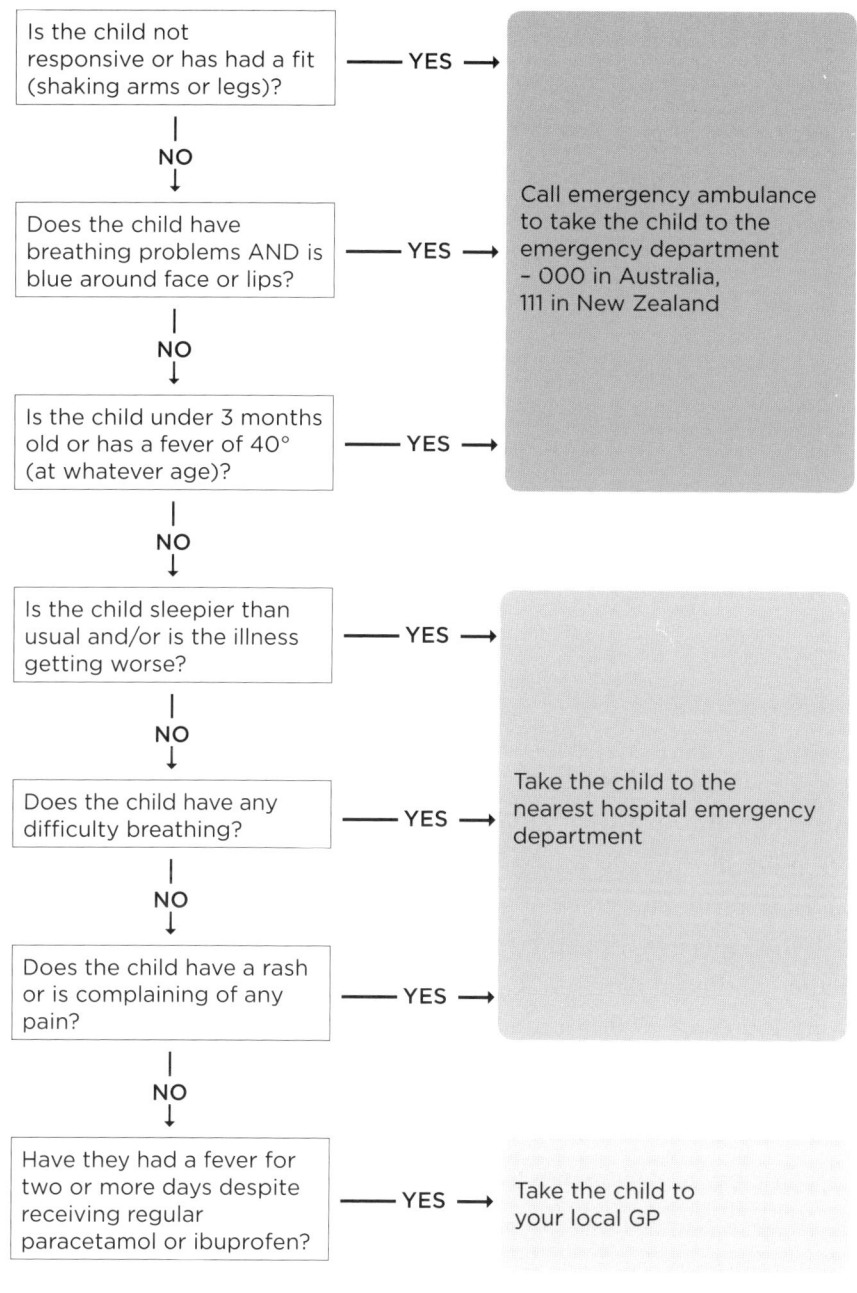

Is the child not responsive or has had a fit (shaking arms or legs)? —— YES →

NO ↓

Does the child have breathing problems AND is blue around face or lips? —— YES →

NO ↓

Is the child under 3 months old or has a fever of 40° (at whatever age)? —— YES →

Call emergency ambulance to take the child to the emergency department - 000 in Australia, 111 in New Zealand

NO ↓

Is the child sleepier than usual and/or is the illness getting worse? —— YES →

NO ↓

Does the child have any difficulty breathing? —— YES →

Take the child to the nearest hospital emergency department

NO ↓

Does the child have a rash or is complaining of any pain? —— YES →

NO ↓

Have they had a fever for two or more days despite receiving regular paracetamol or ibuprofen? —— YES → Take the child to your local GP

7

Breathing Difficulties

Although the majority of illnesses that cause breathing difficulties are mild and usually resolve themselves without hospital admission or long-term effects, they can become serious. They account for half the visits to GPs and 20 to 30 per cent of hospital admissions for acute childhood illnesses. Respiratory illnesses are also the fifth most common cause of death in children between the ages of one and 14. So it is vital to be able to spot when a child is either severely ill or has been mildly ill but is getting worse.

WHAT IS A RESPIRATORY TRACT INFECTION?

Each year, the average preschool child will have five to ten colds. The common cold virus usually causes upper respiratory tract infections (URTIs). A URTI occurs above the vocal cords, which are about midway down the throat. A lower respiratory tract infection (LRTI) is below the vocal cords. The most common LRTI in infants is bronchiolitis which, like the common cold, is caused by a virus.

Croup, recognised by a barking cough, is a URTI. Infections of the respiratory tract are the most frequent cause of breathing difficulties for children.

Pneumonia is an infection of the tissues of the lungs, and it can be caused by either viruses or bacteria. Asthma is a non-infective chronic disease and acute episodes – when wheezing occurs along with fast breathing, a high heart rate and a recurrent or chronic cough – can be extremely serious. Some respiratory illnesses in children are due to problems that may have developed while the child was inside the mother's womb, such as meconium aspiration or inadequate lung development, and some are the result of inherited diseases, such as cystic fibrosis.

As mentioned, most of the respiratory tract infections that cause breathing difficulties in children are not serious, last for only a few days and do not require any specific treatment. Eighty to 90 per cent of these infections are caused by viruses, which can cause several different types of illness. One type of virus, for example, can cause croup, pneumonia and the common cold.

Less commonly, respiratory infections may be due to bacteria, which tend to cause more severe illness. Unlike infections due to viruses, these are usually treated by antibiotics.

HOW BREATHING DIFFICULTIES OCCUR

Children are susceptible to respiratory tract infections because their immune systems are still maturing. As your child gets older, so does their resistance to infection because their immune system

Respiratory infections can be caused by a variety of different bacteria, which may have very different shapes and sizes.

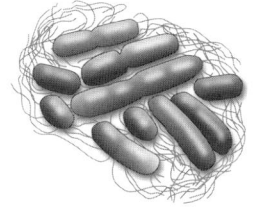
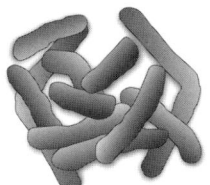
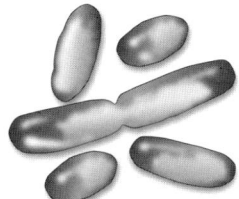

gets better at recognising and fighting off more infectious organisms by producing special cells called antibodies. The body produces one type of antibody for each specific organism, and our bodies can 'remember' each infection and are therefore able to fight them off more effectively (see Chapter 5: Infections).

UPPER RESPIRATORY TRACT INFECTIONS

Approximately 80 per cent of respiratory infections involve just the nose, throat, ears or sinuses, otherwise known as the upper respiratory tract.

The common cold

This is the most common upper respiratory tract infection (see Chapter 5: Infections).

Croup

Croup is a viral infection of the large (upper) airways and it typically affects children aged between six months and five years. It is often characterised by

- several days of high temperature and cold-like symptoms,
- followed by a barking cough, hoarseness and noisy breathing or stridor.

Stridor is the sound heard while the child is breathing in — it may sound high pitched, rasping or squeaking. The more severe the croup the more pronounced the stridor, until the condition is very serious — and the child is extremely ill — when it once again becomes quiet. The symptoms are most severe in children who are younger than three years of age.

Croup is most likely to occur during the winter months and early spring. Only about 3 per cent of children develop croup in each year. A much smaller number have symptoms that continue for up to a week, with fewer than 5 per cent of those infected needing admission to hospital. The symptoms of croup are often worse at night, and this causes a great deal of concern for parents.

TREATMENT

Your doctor may treat moderate cases of croup with one or two doses of a steroid taken orally. This often improves the symptoms significantly. Children with croup who are less than a year old or who do not have easy access to a hospital are more likely to be admitted to hospital for observation, but the majority do not require hospitalisation because the symptoms usually resolve after three or four days. If there are any signs of respiratory distress, and definitely if you can hear stridor while your child is at rest, you should seek a medical opinion.

Whooping cough (pertussis)

Whooping cough is a very contagious infection caused by bacteria called *Bordetella pertussis*. Pertussis means 'forceful cough', and a continuous coughing fit with the 'whoop' sound on breathing in are characteristic symptoms. Whooping cough

- starts with cold-like symptoms,
- is followed by the development of the typical cough, which usually begins at night,
- may cause gagging or vomiting after prolonged coughing episodes.

Whooping cough is potentially deadly and kills many children in third world countries where there is no vaccination program. In recent years it has been on the rise in Australia and New Zealand.

PREVENTION

The most effective way of treating whooping cough is to prevent it by vaccination. While no vaccination is 100 per cent effective, the whooping cough vaccination works in approximately 75 per cent of those immunised against the disease. Side effects from the vaccine are uncommon and minor, such as fevers, swelling and redness at the injection site, so it makes sense to do it. In societies where vaccination levels have fallen, whooping cough is becoming more prevalent. If you have concerns over whether to have your child vaccinated you should discuss this with your GP, and also read the section on immunisation in Chapter 5: Infections (page 77).

TREATMENT

For children who are diagnosed with whooping cough the treatment is antibiotics (usually erythromycin or roxithromycin are used), and even then the symptoms of cough will last a long time. Antibiotics do reduce the period when your child has the potential to spread the disease to others. The cough may last such a long time that in China it is referred to as the '100-day cough'.

LOWER RESPIRATORY TRACT INFECTIONS

The lower respiratory tract is made up of the lung tissues, with the tubes that lie within them and bring them inhaled air. Because the size of the tubes is smaller in younger children and babies, any infection can be potentially serious as they may be more easily blocked.

Bronchiolitis

Bronchiolitis is a viral infection that affects the lungs of younger children, usually babies under the age of one. It is the most common serious respiratory infection of infancy.

The symptoms are:

- fever with a runny nose,
- followed by a period of dry cough, breathlessness and wheeze.

It can be particularly troublesome for children who have other medical problems or were born prematurely, in which case extra care and vigilance are necessary.

Bronchiolitis causes about 1 to 2 per cent of children below the age of 12 months to be admitted to hospital each year, with those most commonly affected aged between two and six months. Bronchiolitis may be severe in very young babies under six weeks and in infants with conditions such as congenital heart disease or chronic lung disease, but most episodes of bronchiolitis are mild and can be managed at home.

TREATMENT

There is no specific cure for bronchiolitis. The treatment is supportive, such as providing oxygen through a mask to make it easier for the child to breathe until their body can fight off the infection. Needing this oxygen therapy means that they will have to stay in the hospital because the medical and nursing staff will want to observe them while they are being treated.

Another common reason that children might be admitted to hospital with bronchiolitis is because the breathlessness prevents them from eating, in which case an intravenous drip may be necessary.

Antibiotics are not effective against viral infections and so usually have no role in the treatment of bronchiolitis.

As with all childhood illnesses, if there is an increase in breathing difficulties, poor pallor, grey-blue lips and/or drowsiness, call the emergency number – 000 in Australia and 111 in New Zealand – for an ambulance to take your child to hospital for immediate medical assessment.

Pneumonia

Pneumonia is an acute infection of the tissues of the lungs, caused by a virus or bacteria. About 3 to 4 per cent of children contract it each year and 150 million are affected worldwide, with a little over 10 per cent of these being admitted to hospital.

Pneumonia is a major cause of hospital admission in children under five years of age; in Auckland, for example, the hospitalisation rate for children under two years old is 11 times the rate for those children over four years old.

Indigenous children are at particular risk – they have a 10 to 20 times higher risk of hospitalisation compared with non-Indigenous children. Indigenous children also spend longer in hospital per episode of the disease and are more likely to have multiple admissions with pneumonia.

Although the death rate from pneumonia in the western world is less than one in 1000, it is the major killer of children worldwide and may account for up to three million deaths per year, or as many as 29 per cent of deaths in the under-five age group.

The symptoms of pneumonia are:

- fever
- cough
- fast breathing rate
- in-drawing or recession of the breastbone
- inability to eat or drink
- cyanosis (blue/grey-coloured lips).

Although most children with pneumonia have coughs and difficulty in breathing, not all children with these signs will have pneumonia. Fever associated with pneumonia is usually above 38°C. Although feeling a child's forehead will not tell you exactly how high the fever is, if their forehead feels cool there is a good chance there is no fever.

The cough may start dry (that is, with no phlegm) but it will usually become loose, and discoloured phlegm is often produced. Seeing phlegm is not necessary for the diagnosis of pneumonia to be considered, since younger children tend not to cough phlegm up.

Children with pneumonia have breathing that is shallow and fast (known as tachypnoea) and they appear afraid to take a deep breath in because of pain. The child will be unwell and lethargic and they may develop sharp pains in the chest. This pain is known as pleurisy, which is caused by the inflammation of the lining of the lung, and it is worse on taking a deep breath in. Younger children may complain of seemingly unrelated symptoms such as abdominal pain and neck stiffness, or simply appear unwell and be off their food.

Definitions of tachypnoea

AGE	BREATHS PER MINUTE
Under 2 months	More than 60
2 to 12 months	More than 50
12 months to 5 years	More than 40

The best predictors of the severity of pneumonia are the rate of breathing and indrawing of the chest wall. In general, a fast breathing rate (see the previous page for age-specific rates), the 'indrawing' of the breastbone, an inability to eat or drink and the appearance of blue/grey-coloured lips (known as cyanosis) are the best signs to tell when a child has low oxygen levels due to pneumonia. A strong relationship has been found between cyanosis, poor feeding and indrawing, and subsequent death.

In its definitions of pneumonia severity the World Health Organization states that, for children up to five years of age, mild pneumonia is characterised by a fast respiratory rate, severe pneumonia by fast breathing and chest wall indrawing, and very severe pneumonia by both of these, along with drowsiness, convulsions or not being able to drink.

For children over the age of five, symptoms are not as predictable. Severity in this age group can still be estimated by a fast breathing rate, high fevers and drowsiness.

WHO definitions of pneumonia severity in children up to five years

	LESS THAN 2 MONTHS OLD	2 MONTHS TO 5 YEARS OLD
Mild pneumonia	Fast breathing rate	Fast breathing rate
Severe pneumonia	Fast breathing rate	Fast breathing rate
	Severe chest wall indrawing	Chest wall indrawing
Very severe pneumonia	Not feeding	Fast breathing rate
	Convulsions	Chest wall indrawing
	Abnormally sleepy or difficult to wake	Drowsiness/convulsions
	Fever/low body temperature	Inability to drink
	Slow irregular breathing	Malnutrition

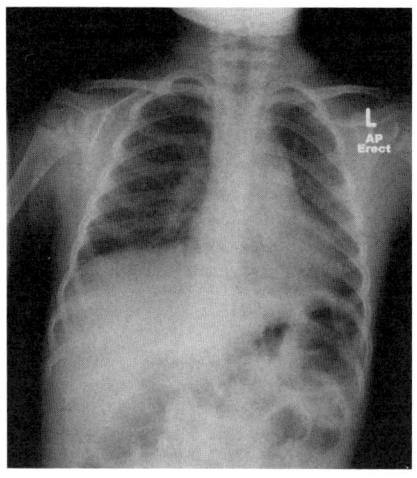

The shadowing in the right lung on this child's x-ray indicates pneumonia.

TREATMENT

Hospital admission for those with pneumonia is often, but not always, required. Antibiotics are usually given, as viral and bacterial pneumonia cannot be reliably differentiated in the early stages. Chest x-rays will be performed, and blood tests (to try to grow bacteria that are causing the disease) may direct treatment in more severe disease.

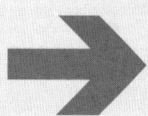

DANGER SIGNS

As children become more ill and exhausted, the earlier signs of fast breathing and the chest wall retracting may disappear. This does not mean that they are getting better, but rather that they are becoming gravely ill and exhausted and need immediate treatment.

Asthma

Asthma is an inflammatory condition of the smaller airways, which results in coughing, wheezing and shortness of breath. It can affect people of all ages. Wheezing in the first two years of a child's life is common and should not necessarily be diagnosed as asthma, as the majority of these children grow out of their symptoms by school age. In fact, although wheezing is often considered the most obvious sign of asthma, it is not always present in children.

Persistent coughing, especially after exercise or at night, may be the most useful sign in helping to diagnose asthma. Infants with asthma often have a cough and rapid breathing, and may also have a large number of 'chest infections'. There may be no obvious wheezing episodes until after 18 to 24 months of age. Shortness of breath and chest tightness may occur alone or in combination with any of the other symptoms and in a young child chest tightness may lead to unexplained irritability. The signs and symptoms of asthma are:

- cough (dry or rattly)
- shortness of breath aggravated by exercise
- wheezing
- chest congestion
- chest tightness
- recurrent bronchitis with croup, bronchiolitis or pneumonia.

The inflammation produced by asthma causes swelling of the lining of the smaller airways, obstructing the flow of air. Air passing through

In those suffering from asthma, inflammation and swelling of the airways causes shortness of breath and wheezing.

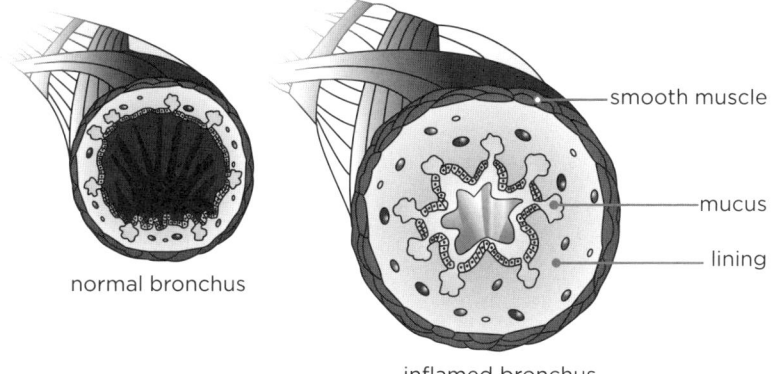

normal bronchus

smooth muscle

mucus

lining

inflamed bronchus

this obstruction causes the wheezy sound typical of asthma, and the extra effort needed to breathe out through narrowed tubes causes fatigue and shortness of breath.

Asthma is the most common chronic (long-term) illness in childhood, and is the most frequent single cause for emergency hospital admission. It affects up to 20 per cent of children and a small proportion of them go on to have asthma as an adult. Asthma may also develop as the child gets older.

Asthma has become increasingly common, although the reasons for this are unclear. The World Health Organization estimates that between 100 and 150 million people worldwide suffer from asthma, and this number is increasing by 50 per cent every ten years. Children exposed to cigarette smoke in the home have an increased incidence of lung infections, asthma and cot death.

There are multiple causes of asthma, and in any one case there are likely to be several factors present. There is certainly an inherited link, as first-degree relatives (close relatives such as brothers, sisters, fathers and mothers) of people with asthma are much more likely to develop asthma. Eczema, hay fever and urticaria (hives) are also associated conditions. There is also a link between asthma and allergy, especially in childhood – which means that if a child has asthma and is allergic to cat fur, for example, the symptoms may be greatly worsened in the presence of cats. The most common cause of worsening asthma symptoms, however, is an infection affecting the upper airways – in other words, a cold 'which goes to the chest'. Exercise, a smoky atmosphere or cold temperatures can bring on the symptoms.

TREATMENT

The treatment of asthma is twofold. Firstly, a drug that opens up the airways such as salbutamol (Ventolin) is usually given in the form of an inhaler (most often through a spacer until the child develops enough coordination to work the inhaler alone – this is often not until the age of seven or eight), although very young children may be given salbutamol syrup.

The use of an inhaler often provides relief for the immediate symptoms within a couple of minutes; however, the effect is relatively short lived, so the inhaler treatment may have to be repeated. These types of inhalers are often known as 'relievers' as they treat the immediate symptoms of an attack.

Additionally, the underlying problem of inflammation of the airways is reduced usually with steroids such as Becotide, Becloforte or Flixotide. These have an anti-inflammatory action and are also usually given via an inhaler (with or without the spacer). Not all children with asthma will need a steroid inhaler. A couple of puffs from a steroid inhaler will not help the immediate problem, but it does have an effect over a period of hours and days. Steroid inhalers should always be taken regularly, as prescribed by a doctor, and if the treatment is effective will help to reduce the frequency and severity of attacks. These are often known as 'preventers', as they reduce the frequency and severity of attacks.

Effective treatment of asthma at home may prevent sudden worsening of symptoms. Because allergy often has a part to play in the development of asthma symptoms, an important part of the treatment of allergic asthma is to avoid things that worsen symptoms, such as dust or animal fur, and treatment should be directed at reducing the effects of allergy.

If a child has symptoms of asthma that are worsening despite 'relieving' treatment, then a medical opinion should be sought urgently because further treatment, such as the use of steroid tablets or syrup, may be required. Many people, including children, carry on taking more and more relievers, hoping that their asthma will settle down, but this often masks the true seriousness of the episode. If your child is not improving despite increasing doses of inhalers, you should take them to the emergency department for assessment.

It's worth working out an 'asthma action plan' with your GP and writing it down so you have a clear idea of what to do at different stages – for example, increasing medications yourself, seeing the GP or going straight to hospital.

After a certain age (around five to six years) a 'peak flow' meter should be used to objectively gauge the degree of the disease. What this allows you to do as a parent is to gauge what your child can blow on the meter when at their best and then what they can do when they are sick. There are standard tables provided so that you can compare these measurements with normal values for children of a certain height, and your GP can then give you an action plan based on actual numbers. This is often a better way of judging asthma severity, rather than what you feel or your child feels, both of which can be far from accurate in gauging the severity of the illness.

Symptoms and signs of worsening asthma

- Breathing that requires increased work
- Intercostal recessions
- Nasal flaring
- Chest pain
- Abnormal breathing pattern, where breathing out takes much longer than breathing in
- Breathing which temporarily stops.

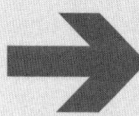

EMERGENCY ASTHMA SYMPTOMS
- Extreme difficulty breathing
- Bluish colour to the lips or face
- Severe anxiety due to shortness of breath
- Rapid pulse
- Sweating
- Decreased level of consciousness (severe drowsiness or confusion) during an attack.

HOW TO RECOGNISE RESPIRATORY DISTRESS

It is vitally important to be able to recognise signs of respiratory distress (breathing difficulties) so you can try and prevent your child becoming more seriously ill. Any child with these symptoms and signs needs immediate medical attention – which may prevent respiratory arrest and death. The degree of the problem will dictate whether and how urgently you need to seek further treatment. You should be vigilant to any indication that symptoms are getting worse in a child.

The signs of respiratory distress

The two key signs of respiratory distress relate to the effort of breathing and the effects of breathing shown by the child.

The effort or work of breathing can be measured by:

- the rate of breathing
- the position the child seeks to adopt
- the use of muscles and movements not usually necessary for breathing
- the noises they make
- how their speech is affected.

The effects of breathing can be gauged by:

- the child's behaviour
- colour
- level of consciousness.

THE EFFORT OF BREATHING

Rate A child's rate of breathing goes up if they are experiencing respiratory distress because they are attempting to get more oxygen into their body to allow it to function properly. However, the normal rate of breathing varies with a child's age, so it can be difficult to work out whether the rate of breathing is abnormal. Ideally, try to have

Normal respiratory rates in children

AGE (in years)	RESPIRATORY RATE (breaths per minute)
1 or under	30–40
1 to 2	25–35
2 to 5	25–30
5 to 12	20–25
Over 12	15–20

one person count the child's respirations for 30 seconds while another person holds them. Multiply the number of respirations by two to get the rate for a minute, which is what any ambulance dispatcher or doctor will need to know. Even more ideal, count the breathing rate for a full minute, but this is often more difficult due to movement.

Sometimes it helps to rest a hand on the chest of the child to feel the movement associated with breathing. With a young child it is useful to try to distract them while you are counting the breathing – because it stops them trying to play with you and preventing your counting and because making it obvious you are counting their breathing may make them hold their breath or breathe differently to normal. A favourite toy may work to distracts them while you count.

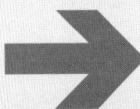

DANGER SIGNS
A rate above 60 breaths per minute is a good indicator of pneumonia and should be taken very seriously. When the child's respiratory rate is high initially, then slows down and is accompanied by lethargy or drowsiness, it is very serious and requires immediate ambulance transfer to an emergency department. Call 000 in Australia, 111 in New Zealand.

Position If a child has respiratory distress they will often try to adopt a position to make their breathing easier and more comfortable. This position should not be forcibly altered.

Often an asthmatic child will sit upright on the side of a bed with their arms outstretched to the sides or in front. This enables the chest wall to provide an anchor for the muscles of their neck and chest to add to the effort of breathing. When a child with respiratory distress tires they may lie down and their effort of breathing may decrease. If this happens spontaneously the child may be exhausted, a very good indicator of severe respiratory distress. A decrease in respiratory distress as a result of effective treatment, on the other hand, is a good thing.

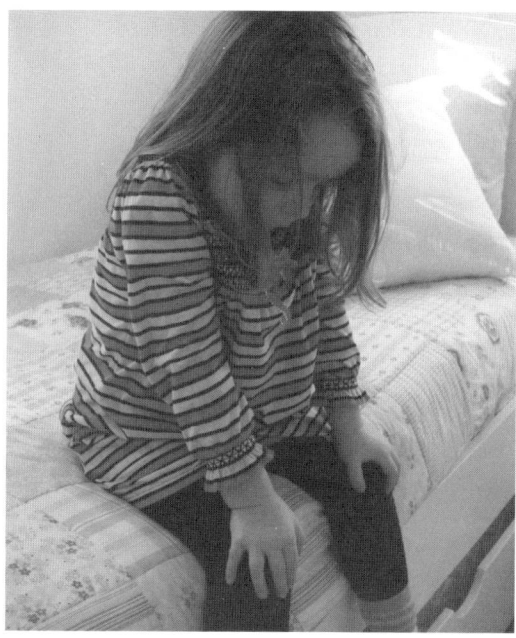

Children who are in respiratory distress will often adopt the 'tripod' position, which helps with breathing.

Muscles and movement A child experiencing respiratory distress may start to use muscles that aren't used when breathing normally. This is indicated by the sucking in of the muscles between the ribs (intercostal), under the ribcage (subcostal) and above the collarbones (supraclavicular), as well as increased use of the muscles at the front and

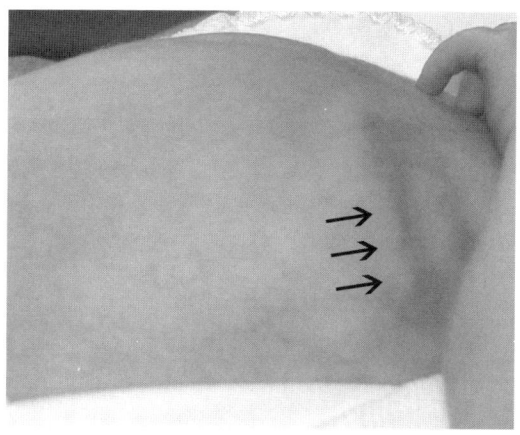

The muscles in the chest between the ribs (the intercostal muscles) contract when a baby is short of breath. This is known as 'intercostal recession' and is a sign of respiratory distress.

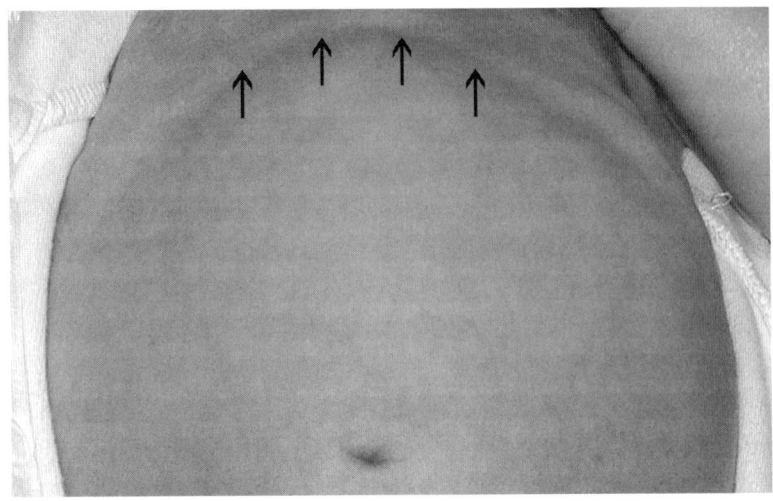

The muscles in the abdomen below the ribs (the subcostal muscles) contract when a baby is short of breath. This is known as 'subcostal recession'.

side of their neck. The breastbone (or sternum) itself may be drawn in with the increased effort of breathing and the nostrils may be flared. In young children and babies 'head nodding' may also occur when the excessive use of the neck muscles to assist breathing exhausts the child so they pull their head down with every breath. These are all signs of respiratory distress and urgent treatment should be sought.

Noises When a child is resting, noises while breathing in such as a rasping noise on breathing in or out indicate significant respiratory distress. In a child with asthma, wheezing usually occurs when breathing out but, contrary to intuition, the noises can decrease when it becomes so severe that they are tired and no longer fighting to breathe.

A loud wheeze does not indicate a serious condition, but the opposite. Decreasing loudness of wheeze, particularly when the child is tiring, means immediate treatment is required. Grunting is also often a sign of extreme respiratory effort, particularly in young children. A child who is grunting while breathing needs immediate medical attention.

Speech If a child is old enough to speak, you should attempt a conversation with them and try to get them to talk in sentences. Not being able to talk in full sentences, only making single-word responses or not making any response at all are increasing signs of the need for immediate medical attention.

THE EFFECTS OF BREATHING

Behaviour Acute breathlessness is a frightening thing for both children and adults, and the child can become very agitated, making it difficult for you to calm them down. Sometimes, although your concerns as parents form an essential part of the medical assessment of your acutely unwell child, these concerns may adversely affect the situation – the fact that you are obviously so worried can make your child more frightened. As a carer, it is important to do all you can to keep everyone as calm as possible to enable effective treatment to be given.

Colour Sometimes the level of oxygen in a child's blood becomes so low during respiratory distress that the haemoglobin in their red blood cells changes from bright red to dark red. This can cause areas where the layer of skin is thin, such as over the lips, to appear darker. The lips and tongue of children who are in extreme respiratory distress may look dusky blue, grey or purple in colour. This is called cyanosis, and it is a sign of imminent collapse and of potential cardiac arrest. Call for an ambulance immediately.

If a child's breathing starts to become very slow and laboured, or if there is a bluish tinge to their skin or lips, these can be signs that things are worsening fast and an ambulance needs to be called for immediate transfer to hospital.

If the child stops breathing, follow the guidelines given in Chapter 24: Basic life support.

Level of consciousness As the levels of oxygen in a person's blood go down, the brain and nervous system start to fail. As well as agitation and distress, this can indicate a decrease in the level of consciousness. A child with severe breathing problems often becomes increasingly drowsy, gradually getting to a point where they cannot be woken. This is a sign of imminent collapse and possible cardiac arrest.

The level of consciousness in children is measured and described by the AVPU scale. The scale enables carers and bystanders not only to estimate the level of consciousness but also, more importantly, to identify and communicate changes.

THE AVPU SCALE

A Alert
V Responds to **V**oice
P Responds to **P**ain
U **U**nresponsive

At the hospital

When you arrive, your child will be assessed and triaged depending on the severity of illness. Asthma is serious and breathing disorders in children often herald severe illness, so you will be placed in a high category, assessed quickly and treatment started within a short period of time. Always attempt to give a clear, concise history – this will help staff diagnose the problem and judge the severity of the illness.

If your child has been working very hard at breathing and then appears to be quiet or have a decreased level of consciousness, this could indicate an extremely severe illness and an immediate threat to life, so ensure the staff recognise this and give treatment immediately.

An important part of assessing your child's progress is the pulse oximeter applied to their finger, ear lobe or forehead, which measures the oxygen in the blood, but also important is your perception of progress so you must keep the staff aware if you believe there is any deterioration or if you think there is no improvement.

Treatment may include oxygen and drugs given through spacers or nebulisers to help with asthma, even if your child has no history of asthma (it may be the first episode). Although asthma is not generally diagnosed in children under two years of age, puffers with spacers are still attempted as they sometimes help and may also indicate airways that are prone to be 'reactive', or to show wheeze and other asthma symptoms when inflamed or infected.

Chest x-rays are commonly given in asthma, but are not always useful. They should be performed in order to make a specific diagnosis (such as pneumonia) or to direct treatment, not just to confirm a diagnosis. In asthma they are very rarely required and seldom change the management of the illness – no child who is severely ill should be moved out of an emergency department to an x-ray department for this investigation.

Antibiotics are often overused by GPs and doctors in hospitals. They are often given because of a perceived parental desire so it is important to ask the medical staff for clarification of the need for such treatment – indeed, for the reasons why any medication is given.

If your child is being discharged, be sure you have a clear idea of what you are being advised to do and when, and who is going to review them and when. Make sure you have the necessary prescriptions and that you can get to a pharmacy to fill them. Dealing with a severely sick child is a very harrowing experience for all concerned, so don't expect to remember all the instructions. Ask the staff to write them down for you as part of an asthma action plan.

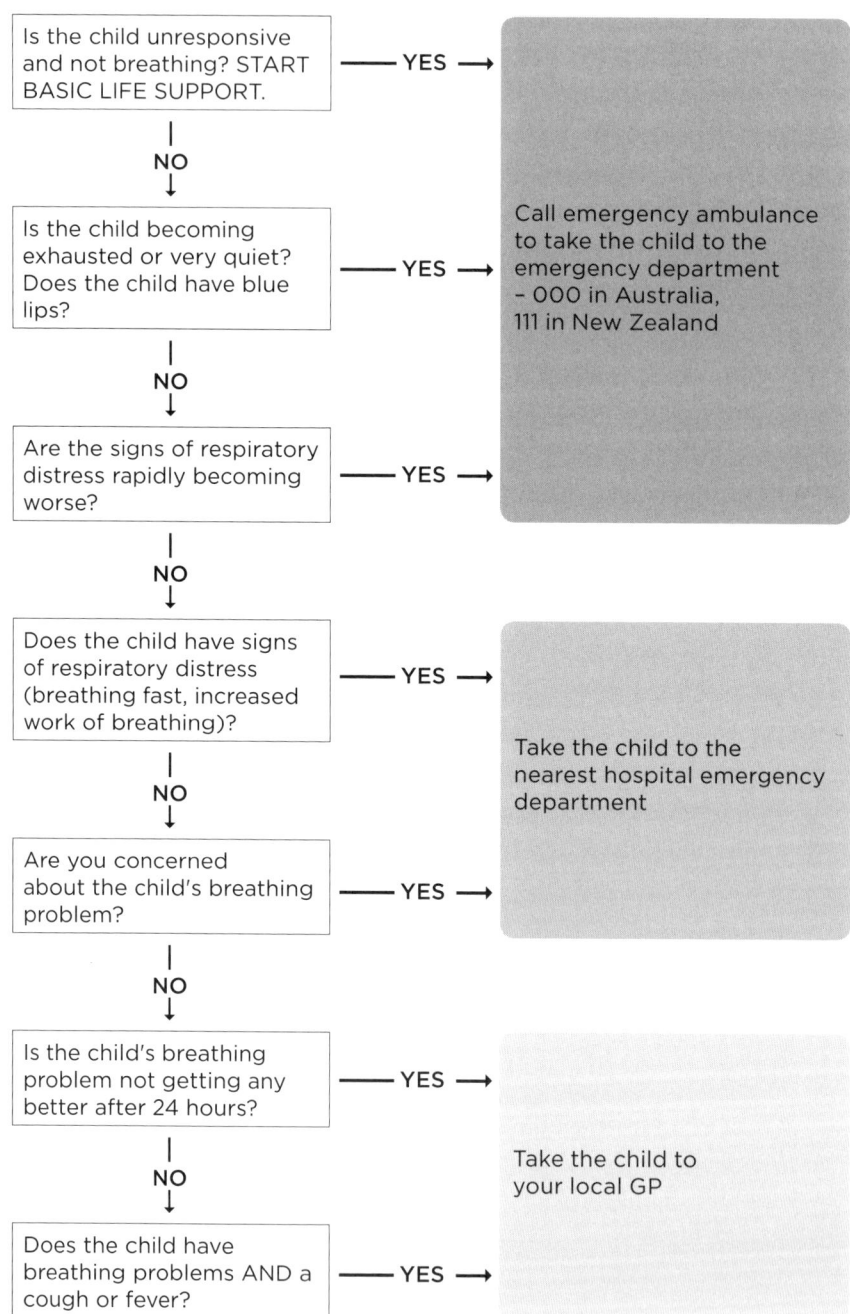

Is the child unresponsive and not breathing? START BASIC LIFE SUPPORT.

— YES →

NO ↓

Is the child becoming exhausted or very quiet? Does the child have blue lips?

— YES →

Call emergency ambulance to take the child to the emergency department – 000 in Australia, 111 in New Zealand

NO ↓

Are the signs of respiratory distress rapidly becoming worse?

— YES →

NO ↓

Does the child have signs of respiratory distress (breathing fast, increased work of breathing)?

— YES →

Take the child to the nearest hospital emergency department

NO ↓

Are you concerned about the child's breathing problem?

— YES →

NO ↓

Is the child's breathing problem not getting any better after 24 hours?

— YES →

Take the child to your local GP

NO ↓

Does the child have breathing problems AND a cough or fever?

— YES →

8

ABDOMINAL PAIN

Abdominal pain is one of the most common reasons parents take children to GPs and emergency departments. When a child complains of abdominal pain, they could have a trivial or a life-threatening condition. The causes of abdominal pain in a child are often difficult to tease out and can only be assessed in the overall context of the history taken by the parents, what the child is able to describe, the examination by the doctor and laboratory results. An older child can often give a clear description of the pain that can be very useful.

WHAT CAUSES ABDOMINAL PAIN?

There are many causes, but the best way to think of them is in five distinct groups. This allows the problem to seem less complex.

Infectious gastroenteritis This is most commonly caused by viruses or bacteria. Organisms called protozoa, parasites such as giardia and worms may also be the cause of the pain.

Surgical problems This is a term used by doctors to describe a multitude of issues that have traditionally been dealt with by surgery. These include appendicitis and all the things that can block or obstruct the bowel.

Food and digestion related This includes food poisoning, allergic reactions to foods, and gastric and bowel distension. The food poisoning here is slightly different from that discussed in Chapter 5: Infections (see page 68), because the infecting organism makes a toxin outside the body and that toxin causes the symptoms, which are usually short lived. Pain in the gastric and bowel areas from gas (blowing up) may be called colic; however, colic is difficult to accurately define. It really refers to a type of abdominal pain that is centred around the belly button and gets worse in spasms at regular intervals.

Poisons or toxins These might have been ingested by the patient either by mistake or deliberately as part of self-harm. It could be in the form of iron tablets, paracetamol or alcohol. Also included in this group are bites from spiders and snakes.

Problems outside the digestive system These medical issues may arise in the lungs or the bladder, for instance. Problems such as diabetes (caused by the body's inability to control sugar), pneumonia, urinary tract infection, testicular torsion (twisting) and hip problems can all cause abdominal pain. In reality, a child may also complain of abdominal pain with any systemic illness.

For doctors to diagnose exactly what might be causing the problem, the key clues are other symptoms and signs that may occur with the abdominal pain – that is, how fast the pain came on, where in the abdomen it is felt, whether the pain seems to go anywhere else, and if anything makes it better or worse. All of the conditions causing abdominal pain are listed on the opposite page, with the other symptoms that may help to pinpoint which conditions your child is suffering from.

CAUSES OF ABDOMINAL PAIN IN CHILDREN

Appendicitis: pain starting in the centre and moving to the right lower abdomen.

Bowel obstruction: vomiting and abdominal distension (swelling).

Pancreatitis: severe pain felt at the front that 'radiates' to the back, feeling as if it goes straight through the body.

Trauma: bruising, grazing or cuts to the abdominal wall.

Gastroenteritis, with vomiting and diarrhoea: usually after close contact with someone with similar symptoms.

Parasitic infection, with diarrhoea, loss of weight.

Urinary tract infection: pain on passing water, weeing more often, wetting pants/the bed.

Diabetes, with vomiting and dehydration.

Inflammatory bowel disease, with diarrhoea with blood or mucus, and previous episodes of the same symptoms.

Torsion of the testicle: sudden very painful testicle and vomiting.

Constipation: decreased bowel movements and swelling of abdomen.

Lower lobe pneumonia: cough producing yellow or green spit.

Hernia: painful swelling in the groin area.

Diagnosing abdominal pain

Whereas infants will simply be irritable and off their food and toddlers may get angry and behave differently, schoolage children often complain of abdominal pain to either get your attention or to alert you to a life-threatening condition. There can seem to be no apparent distinction. An older child or teenager may not report pain immediately, depending on their social schedule or what they perceive as a risk of embarrassment.

Despite all this, there are clear pointers or red flags to serious illness that you should look out for.

Onset Note whether the pain come on suddenly or was associated with a particular activity such as eating (which would imply infected food, digestion problems or possibly a surgical problem). A more gradual onset could be caused by any of the conditions listed on page 107. Other associated conditions, with symptoms described as 'just diarrhoea' or 'worse before meals', may point to gastroenteritis (infection) or gastritis (inflammation of the stomach), respectively.

Duration Any pain is potentially a serious problem but a doctor must definitely review prolonged or ongoing pain. Even if your child appears well and the pain seems minor, if it hasn't gone away after about 12 to 24 hours, they must be seen. If the pain is severe and/or they appear unwell, then you should see a doctor immediately.

Location and migration Most pain is initially described as central (around the belly button). If this settles and your child appears well in a very short time, it is probably not significant. However, if the pain migrates to the right lower abdomen it indicates appendicitis. This is even more likely if the pain started in the right lower abdomen (which a doctor would still consider as a possible appendicitis until proven otherwise).

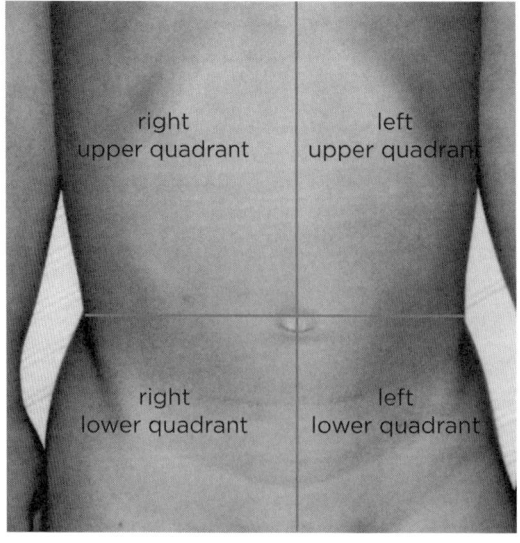

right
upper quadrant

left
upper quadrant

right
lower quadrant

left
lower quadrant

A child's abdomen divided into the four quadrants. Doctors divide the abdomen into these quadrants as a way to describe the location of pain.

When boys locate pain anywhere in their abdomen you should also think about possible testicle problems, such as torsion (twisting), especially if they complain of groin pain. Be highly suspicious that it might be torsion, as the twisting of the spermatic cord that connects to the testicles can cut off the blood supply and result in the complete loss of the testicle in a very short time. Lower abdominal pain with or without urinary symptoms could be due to a urinary tract infection.

General appearance If the child appears unwell, is sweating and pale, or you are concerned for any other reason you cannot precisely describe, seek medical help urgently.

Vomiting This may not signal a serious problem, but any vomiting that is yellow or green (bile) or blood stained or which occurs persistently immediately on or after eating needs medical attention (see Chapter 9: Vomiting and diarrhoea).

Fever This may be associated with a viral gastroenteritis but it could also be caused by a urinary tract infection, which is a condition that requires medical attention due to its potential to damage the kidneys, especially in young children. It is not always easy to distinguish

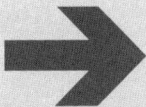

DANGER SIGNS
- Central abdominal pain that settles in the right lower quadrant
- Severe pain, especially if your child draws the legs up to the chest
- Persistent pain, especially if associated with other 'systemic' symptoms, such as cough, temperature, dehydration, etc.
- Sudden onset of severe pain.

Any pain other than temporary pain and in a well child should be considered as potentially serious.

between these symptoms so any child with abdominal pain and fever should be seen by a doctor and a urine sample taken, as detecting early urinary tract infections can prevent the damage to the kidney that occurs with recurrent infections.

Rash Any rash with abdominal pain may herald serious illness and you should see a doctor immediately.

Contacts If others in your family, your child's friends or schoolmates are affected by the same symptom, it probably implies an infective source or possibly food poisoning.

SOME COMMON ABDOMINAL PAIN PROBLEMS
Appendicitis
The appendix is a small pouch of bowel about the size of a short, fat worm, and if it becomes infected or inflamed it causes appendicitis. The pain from appendicitis typically (but not always) starts around the tummy button, then moves to the right lower quadrant of the abdomen. Affected children usually have a fever, feel nauseated, vomit and tend not to want to eat or drink.

The appendix is located in the right lower quadrant. It can become inflamed, a condition that is known as appendicitis, causing abdominal pain.

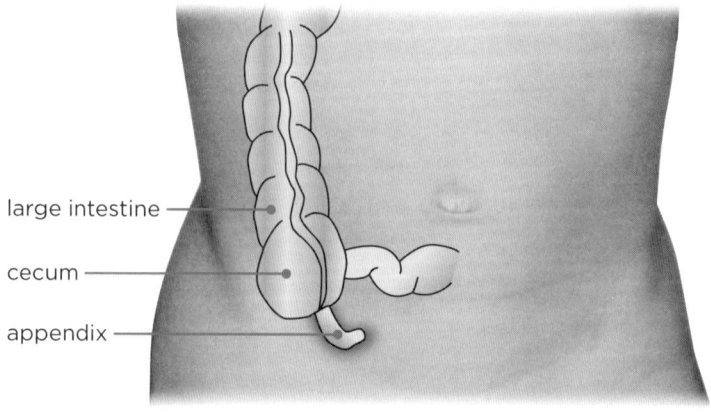

large intestine

cecum

appendix

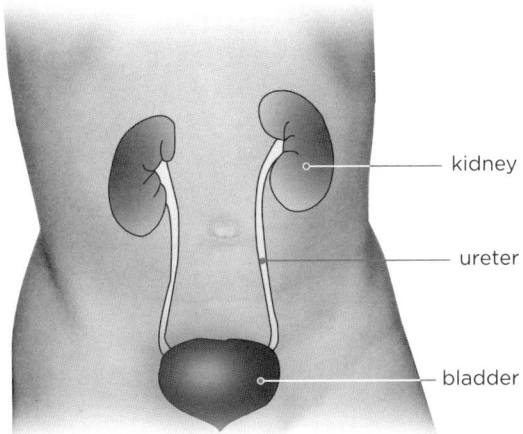

Infections of the kidneys, ureters and bladder are known as urinary tract infections and are treated with antibiotics.

kidney

ureter

bladder

TREATMENT

Often an ultrasound scan will be needed to confirm the diagnosis. The treatment for appendicitis is the surgical removal of the appendix, an operation that is called an appendicectomy.

Urinary tract infections

Infections of the bladder or kidneys are common in children. These are collectively known as urinary tract infections (or UTIs).

The symptoms of a UTI can vary from child to child. The majority will have mild symptoms but some can develop signs of a severe infection and will need to be admitted to hospital.

Older children may complain of abdominal pain, fever and they may exhibit signs such as wetting themselves, having pain when weeing or going to the toilet more often than they do normally. Infants and babies will generally be irritable with vomiting and a fever.

TREATMENT

UTIs are diagnosed by analysing a sample of the child's urine. The treatment is a course of antibiotics.

Most children with a UTI will require a follow-up consultation with a specialist (a paediatrician) to check for any underlying problems with their kidneys or bladder.

Colic

Colic is often talked about and it can be challenging and difficult for doctors and parents alike, and frustrating and very tiring for families. It is a common condition, occurring in about one in every ten babies. Colic is defined as an attack of sudden crying and apparent abdominal pain in early infancy. It is characterised by episodes of irritability, loud crying and what appears to be abdominal pain (when the baby draws up their legs and their abdomen feels rigid). Other typical features of a colic episode include being usually associated with feeding and coming on suddenly. The baby appears upset and their crying is loud. They may take up to four hours to settle. There can be apparent abdominal distension (increase in the size of the abdomen), although this may be difficult to assess.

There are many and varied theories regarding the causes of colic, but often there are clear dietary issues such as sensitivity or allergies to certain foods. Colic is a problem experienced by children just several weeks old up to four years of age. There is no evidence that it has any long-term adverse effects.

TREATMENT

As with all recurrent pain, it is very important to treat each episode on its own merits. Any deviation from the norm should be treated with suspicion – this will often be apparent with so-called 'colicky' babies, as the regularity of the problem is characteristic and tiring to parents, so anything out of the ordinary will be noted. Once an initial assessment to exclude serious and specific conditions has been carried out, the usual approach is to wait until the pain goes, watching to make sure that no symptoms of other illnesses appear.

Recurrent pain

Recurrent abdominal pain is one of the most common symptoms in childhood worldwide. It is responsible for missed school days, a high use of health resources and of considerable morbidity (further problems caused by illness). It can be caused by both functional and organic disorders (functional disorders are those not explained by organic medical problems; organic means disorders that can be diagnosed, given the current state of medical knowledge, skill and technology).

The management and diagnosis of these disorders is beyond the scope of this book but the key point to be aware of is that even in children who have recurrent abdominal pain, serious and life-threatening conditions can still occur which may or may not be related to the recurrent problem.

Children with recurrent pain should be seen regularly by their GP and have whatever tests are felt to be appropriate. Some may need referral to a paediatric gastroenterologist or to a paediatrician. Episodes that are different from those previously observed should be taken seriously, and consultation with the treating physician or in a hospital emergency department is essential if you are concerned. Despite the difficulty in identifying the cause for a lot of recurrent pain, a child should never be treated as if they are 'crying wolf'. If you are vigilant you will not miss episodes that are significant. If there is any doubt then consult your doctor.

At the doctor's

As abdominal pain is often difficult to assess in all ages and may herald severe disease, it is common for a child to have various tests when visiting the doctor or hospital. However, with persistent pain, a clinical examination, especially if performed by an experienced doctor and repeated over a few hours, remains the best tool for gauging if there is a serious problem.

For pain that improves by itself (called 'self-limiting') and when a normal examination has taken place, no further action may be required.

Urine tests should be mandatory in any child with abdominal pain, as urinary tract infections are common and are serious if missed in children. Blood tests are often performed and they may give a non-specific picture of inflammation which could be present in the body – for the most part they cannot rule in or rule out a particular disease or surgical problem.

Occasionally x-rays are used for abdominal pain, and these may be useful if there is any possibility of a blockage or obstruction to the bowel. They would often be performed if there is a suspicion that your child has swallowed a foreign body. Ultrasound uses soundwaves to form a picture of tissues deep in the abdomen and can be a very good diagnostic tool. A CT scan may be useful for diagnosis, although it gives a substantial radiation dose and will be avoided if possible. The risks and benefits must be weighed up by your physician and discussed with you before its use.

TREATMENT

The treatment will depend wholly on the diagnosis made when you go to the doctor. Should the pain settle quickly, and your child appears well and is eating and drinking without problems, then nothing needs to be done.

If the suspected diagnosis is gastroenteritis, most often this is caused by a virus and other people will be affected in a time period that implies passage from person to another. When everybody in a group or a family gets sick at one time, this would indicate an external infection source or food contaminated with toxins. If your child appears well and you are able to keep them hydrated or re-hydrate them with fluids via the mouth (see Chapter 9: Vomiting and diarrhoea), then following a doctor's advice and treating at home is appropriate.

Any deterioration in your child's condition from a previously stable state should be treated with concern, including any inability to re-hydrate adequately. You should promptly return them to your doctor or the hospital. And remember, no doctor, nurse or paramedic should criticise you for seeking help with a sick child.

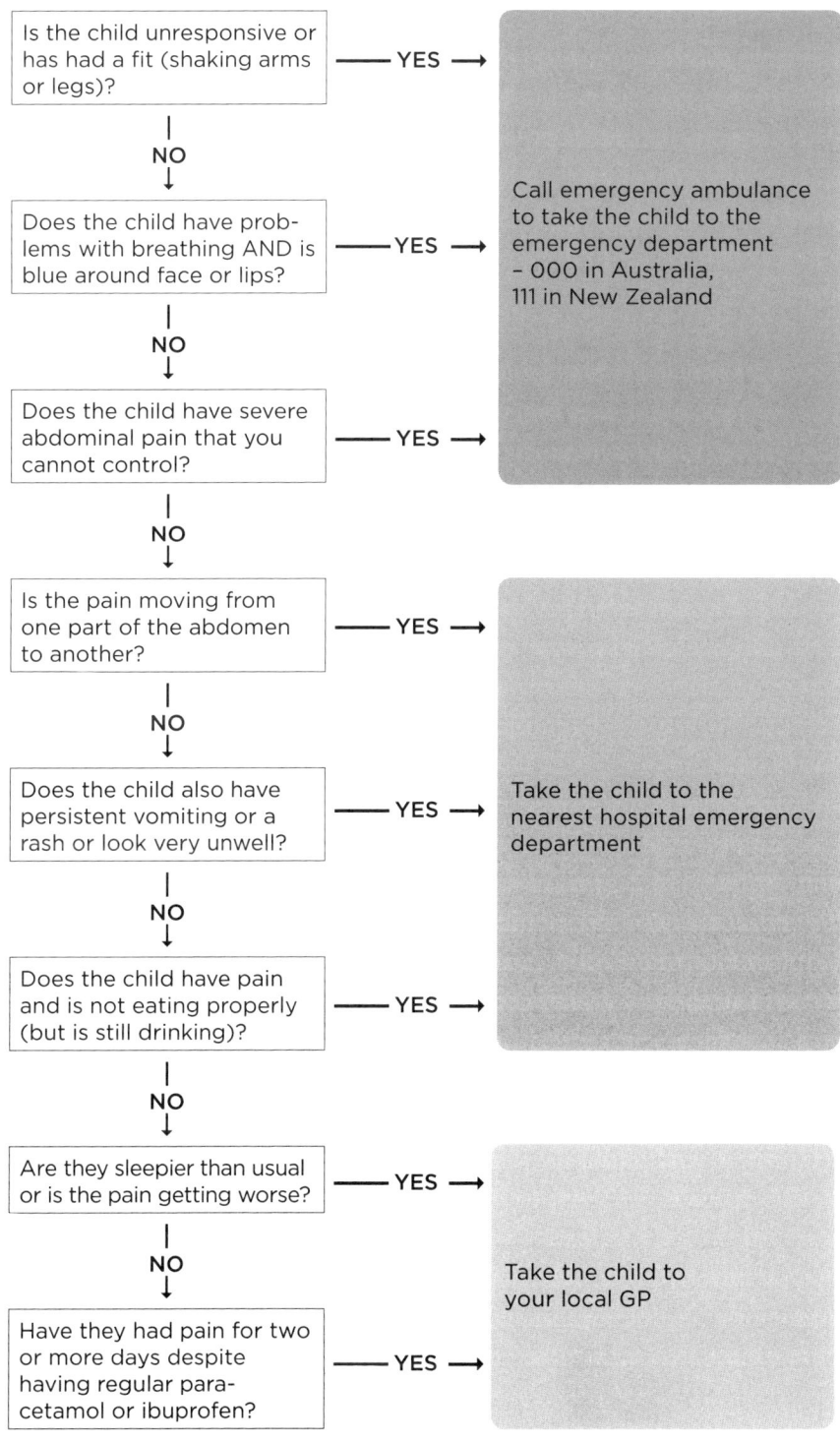

Is the child unresponsive or has had a fit (shaking arms or legs)? —— YES →

NO ↓

Does the child have problems with breathing AND is blue around face or lips? —— YES →

NO ↓

Does the child have severe abdominal pain that you cannot control? —— YES →

Call emergency ambulance to take the child to the emergency department – 000 in Australia, 111 in New Zealand

NO ↓

Is the pain moving from one part of the abdomen to another? —— YES →

NO ↓

Does the child also have persistent vomiting or a rash or look very unwell? —— YES →

Take the child to the nearest hospital emergency department

NO ↓

Does the child have pain and is not eating properly (but is still drinking)? —— YES →

NO ↓

Are they sleepier than usual or is the pain getting worse? —— YES →

NO ↓

Take the child to your local GP

Have they had pain for two or more days despite having regular paracetamol or ibuprofen? —— YES →

9

VOMITING AND DIARRHOEA

It is common for children of any age to suffer an upset tummy with vomiting and/or diarrhoea at one time or another without any serious consequences. The most common cause is gastroenteritis. However, there are many different causes for both conditions and it is important to recognise potentially serious problems – particularly dehydration – that can arise from them.

Most episodes of vomiting and diarrhoea last for only a few days, do not need any specific treatment and do not have any serious consequences. But more serious disorders can lead to poor digestion of food, and this can cause growth and development problems if the situation is not treated. Acute (short-term) disorders do not cause these problems. But in a minority of cases, vomiting and diarrhoea can lead to a more severe illness as a result of loss of fluids and salts.

Vomiting can occur for any number of reasons not related to the gastrointestinal tract, and at times it is an important sign when determining the severity of a child's illness.

GASTROENTERITIS

Gastroenteritis is an inflammation of the stomach and intestines that causes vomiting and diarrhoea. Worldwide, three to five billion cases of gastroenteritis occur every year, predominantly in developing countries as result of poor hygiene and living conditions. Of these, there are around two million deaths in those under five years of age. In developed countries death from gastroenteritis is rare; however, significant and serious consequences can occur from dehydration and irregular levels of salts in the blood as a result of vomiting and diarrhoea.

Around 20 per cent of consultations to GPs in the under fives are for gastroenteritis, and of these about 1 in 20, or 5 per cent, will need to be admitted to hospital. The peak age for infection is six months to two years because of greater risk of faecal-to-oral contamination or spreading through coughing.

CAUSES OF GASTROENTERITIS
Viruses: 70 per cent
Bacteria: 10 to 20 per cent
Protozoa: less than 10 per cent
Helminths (worms): less than 1 per cent

SEVERE SYMPTOMS

When your child is suffering from gastroenteritis, your key objectives are to recognise if they are dehydrated or if at risk of becoming dehydrated, and to determine which features, including vomiting and diarrhoea, may point to a serious underlying disease requiring immediate attention.

Dehydration

Having performed a general assessment of your child's illness (see Chapter 4: How to recognise a seriously ill child), there are some specific pointers which should become apparent if the child is suffering from dehydration.

The most accurate assessment of mild dehydration is a loss of weight over a few days. Other evidence of fluid loss includes:

- absence of tears
- dry lips and tongue
- depressed fontanelle (the hole on the top of the head in infants under 12 months)
- baggy, loose-feeling skin
- decreased urination, which can be determined by either a reduced number and/or weight of nappies in a day, or small volumes of dark urine in older children.

Any change in the child's level of consciousness indicates potentially severe dehydration. Initially the child may seem anxious or agitated and, as dehydration worsens, may become sleepy or difficult to rouse. This is a serious problem and needs urgent attention – call 000 in Australia, 111 in New Zealand. The World Health Organization has developed a system to classify dehydration.

CLASSIFICATIONS FOR DEHYDRATION
No dehydration: Not enough signs to classify as some or severe dehydration.

Some dehydration: Two of the following signs:
- restless, irritable
- sunken eyes
- thirsty, drinks eagerly
- pinched skin returns to normal slowly.

Severe dehydration: Two of the following signs:
- lethargic or unconscious
- sunken eyes
- not able to drink, or drinking poorly
- pinched skin returns to normal very slowly.

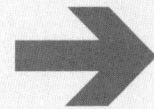

VOMITING: DANGER SIGNS
- Increasing frequency of vomiting
- No appetite
- Bile-coloured vomit
- Blood in vomit
- Vomiting with ongoing pain or distress
- Unable to swallow food
- Any suspicion of poisons
- Projectile vomiting in infants (particularly occurring with little or no notice).

Vomiting

Children vomit for many reasons. Other symptoms can help establish if the vomiting is significant, and in diagnosing an underlying problem.

Symptoms and causes of vomiting

SYMPTOM	DIAGNOSIS
Abdominal pain and diarrhoea	Gastroenteritis
Pain moving from around belly button to right lower abdomen	Appendicitis (see page 110)
Pain and increased frequency of passing urine	Urinary tract infection (see page 111)
Headache, neck stiffness and rash	Meningitis (see page 129)
Abdominal pain, diarrhoea and previous episodes of the same symptoms	Food allergy
Fevers	Fever (see Chapter 6)
Cough, producing coloured spit and breathing problems	Pneumonia (see page 89)
Abdominal pains, breathing problems in a child with diabetes	Diabetes
Head or abdominal injuries	Trauma (see Chapter 18)

Diarrhoea

Diarrhoea can be defined as a stool (poo) that is more liquid than normal and is passed more frequently. It is most often associated with viral gastroenteritis but may be caused by bacterial infection, in which case it may have blood in it. Parasites such as giardia or worms may be the cause; food intolerances and ingestion of poisons or inappropriate medicines should also be considered. Occasionally it can be 'overflow diarrhoea', where a child is constipated and only fluid can move past the mass of faeces contained higher in the bowel, although this is relatively uncommon compared with infective causes. The presence of blood or mucus in the stool may indicate inflammatory bowel disease or infections that need treating with antibiotics.

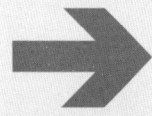

DIARRHOEA: DANGER SIGNS
- Increasing or constant diarrhoea, especially after three days
- Blood and mucus in the diarrhoea
- Severe pain, especially not resolved with a bowel motion.

TREATMENT OF VOMITING AND DIARRHOEA

The use of antibiotics, anti-diarrhoeal medications and antiemetics (anti-nausea medications) are generally not recommended for children, although recently some institutions have been using more antiemetics for children over one year. For the vast majority of vomiting and diarrhoea cases, increasing fluid intake and gradually returning to a normal diet is all that is required. Oral re-hydration supplements (ORS), which have been especially formulated to contain the correct amount of salt and sugar, are beneficial and are available over the counter at any pharmacy. There are some basic principles about re-hydration and a return to a normal diet:

- Infants should be given small sips of water (about 15 millilitres) every five minutes, even if they are still vomiting, and after two hours similar amounts of ORS – children who are vomiting will still tend to keep down more than they lose. If the infant is being breast fed, continue to breast feed and give small sips of water in between, changing to ORS after an hour or so.

- When the symptoms of vomiting settle (this can sometimes happen as the child re-hydrates), often within 6 to 24 hours, the child can restart their normal diet (formula for those using it) but avoid fatty and high sugar foods, and focus more on complex foods such as vegetables.
- In older children, allow their thirst to determine their fluid intake but restrict large amounts of one type of drink – that is, start with water for two hours and then go on to ORS, before resuming a normal diet 12 to 24 hours later.
- Sugary drinks, carbonated drinks, sports drinks, fruit juices, watered-down lemonade and fatty foods are not beneficial and, indeed, may do harm due to the incorrect ratios of sugars and salts for absorption.

If the above measures fail, your child may need to go to hospital to have fluids given intravenously (IV) through a drip or down a feeding tube from the nose into the stomach (via a nasogastric [NG] tube). In acute diarrhoea, medications are not routinely used.

Antibiotics can often make things worse (increase abdominal pain and diarrhoea) and should not be administered unless there is a specific treatable cause – in the form of a bacterium or other organism (such as giardia) – which has been identified by laboratory testing of a faeces sample.

At the doctor's

If your child looks very dehydrated or has some abdominal pain, they may be given priority and seen quickly. If they look well and are not distressed they may have to wait to be seen after more urgent cases are dealt with. Always attempt to give a clear and concise history of the problem to the medical personnel. This might be difficult if you are very worried about your child and preoccupied, but it will help the staff diagnose the problem and judge the severity of the illness.

Your child will be examined and have some tests performed – usually pulse and respiratory rate, and oxygen levels (involving a small probe on their finger or foot). A clinical examination, especially when repeated over a few hours, remains the best tool for gauging if there is a serious problem. Tests may be necessary – including urine tests (to rule out urinary tract infections), blood tests (to look at the salts and infective markers in the blood) and stool sample examinations (a sample of your child's faeces that can be analysed for infection).

If your child is thought to be dehydrated they may be given a 'trial of oral fluids', which consists of small volumes of a salt–and–sugar drink taken regularly. If they are not able to tolerate this, they may need an IV drip to get some fluids into a vein. In this case, they will need to stay in the hospital until they come off the drip.

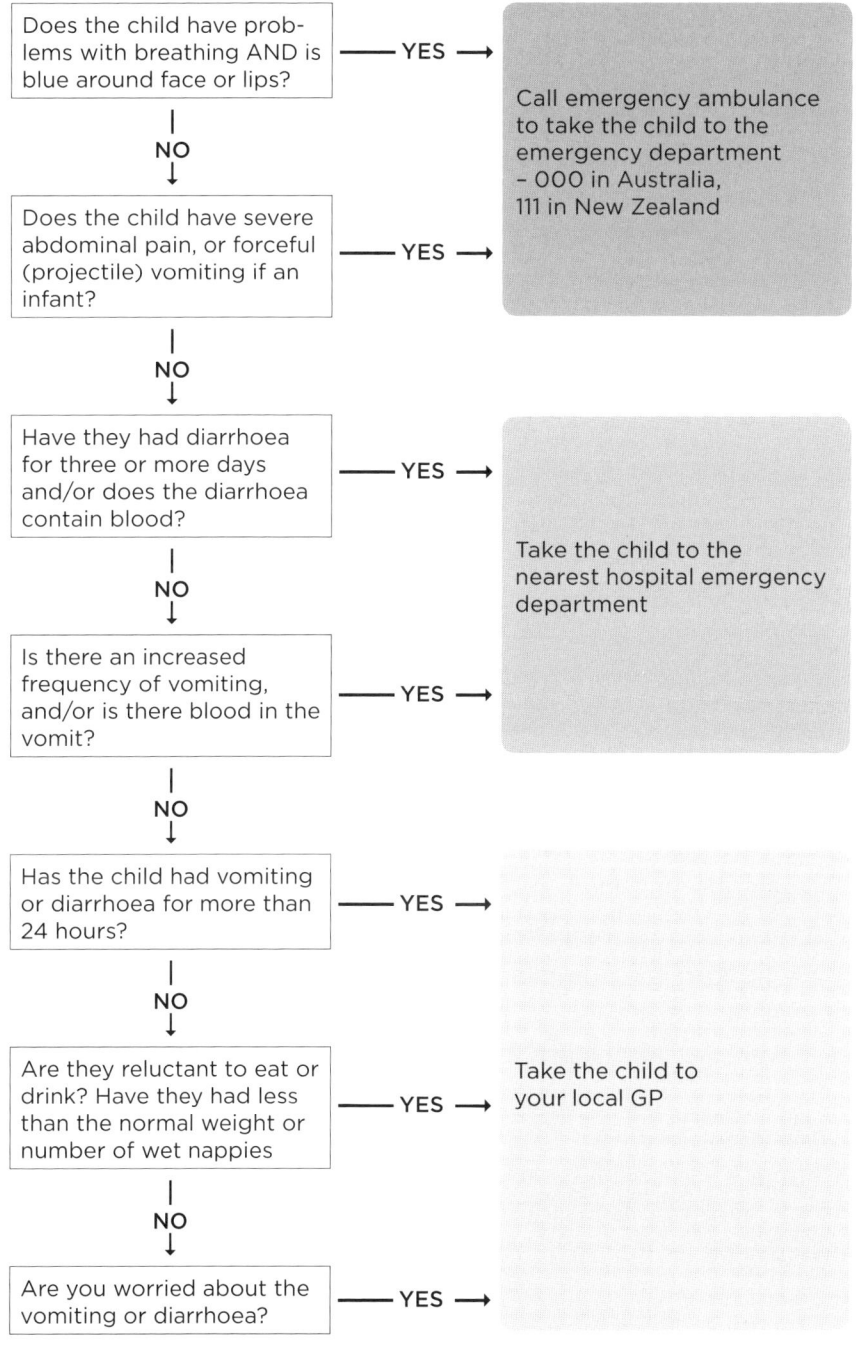

Does the child have problems with breathing AND is blue around face or lips? —— YES →

NO ↓

Does the child have severe abdominal pain, or forceful (projectile) vomiting if an infant? —— YES →

Call emergency ambulance to take the child to the emergency department – 000 in Australia, 111 in New Zealand

NO ↓

Have they had diarrhoea for three or more days and/or does the diarrhoea contain blood? —— YES →

NO ↓

Is there an increased frequency of vomiting, and/or is there blood in the vomit? —— YES →

Take the child to the nearest hospital emergency department

NO ↓

Has the child had vomiting or diarrhoea for more than 24 hours? —— YES →

NO ↓

Are they reluctant to eat or drink? Have they had less than the normal weight or number of wet nappies —— YES →

Take the child to your local GP

NO ↓

Are you worried about the vomiting or diarrhoea? —— YES →

10

FAINTS AND FITS

Faints and fits are both fairly common symptoms in children of any age. Sometimes it is difficult to distinguish between a faint and a fit as they may appear quite alike. There are many causes of both fits and faints. Potentially serious problems are those like meningitis, which need immediately medical attention. The priority for the first aid treatment of conditions that cause fits and faints are assessment and management of the airways, breathing and circulation (see page 252).

Seizures or convulsions in childhood may be the result of a high temperature, epilepsy or a generalised illness and the airway must be kept open and breathing and circulation monitored until the seizure stops. These simple measures can prevent catastrophic complications that may otherwise occur.

FAINTING

A faint is an episode of temporary loss of consciousness followed by a spontaneous and full recovery. The medical term for a faint is syncope. The duration of unconsciousness is rarely more than 20 to 30 seconds.

The reason for fainting is usually a reduction in blood (carrying oxygen) to the brain. Most of us have probably experienced this sensation at some time – it often occurs if we stand up too quickly after sitting or lying down. Collapsing or falling to the ground causes blood to return to the brain, so you regain consciousness.

Sometimes it is difficult to tell if a child has had a fit or a faint. This is because even with faints a child can have some jerking or twitching of the arms and legs.

The features that make it more likely that a fit occurred are:

- loss of consciousness for more than 30 seconds
- biting of the tongue or lips
- being incontinent (wetting their pants)
- being confused or dazed while recovering.

Causes of fainting

Most causes of fainting in children are not serious or life threatening. Approximately 10 to 20 per cent of all children will suffer at least one episode of fainting. Usually a faint occurs because of a stimulus reducing the blood flow to the brain.

Some causes of fainting in childhood include:

- standing up too quickly from lying or sitting down (called an orthostatic syncope)
- minor trauma or pain
- seeing blood on, or trauma to, someone else
- physiological or reflex syncope – for instance, fainting while:
    - stretching or yawning (stretch syncope)
    - coughing forcefully (cough syncope)
    - having a wee (micturition syncope)
    - having a poo (defecation syncope)
    - chewing (deglutition syncope)
    - brushing own hair (hair groomer's syncope)
    - hyperventilation or panic attack.

HEART-RELATED FAINTING

Fainting episodes that occur while a child is doing a physical activity or exerting themselves (running, swimming or playing sports) can sometimes be due to a heart condition – heart-related fainting. So if any such episodes occur, it is vitally important that you take the child to a doctor or to the hospital to get checked. This is because there may be an underlying heart condition that could potentially be life threatening if not recognised and treated.

INITIAL TREATMENT OF FAINTING

Keep your child lying down until they feel better. If they are drowsy or sleepy, put them into the recovery position (see opposite and page 262). If they are unconscious and/or unresponsive, then follow the ABC assessment as described in Chapter 24, Basic life support.

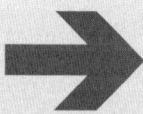

DANGER SIGNS
- Fainting during exercise or exertion
- Loss of consciousness with a head injury
- Loss of consciousness for more than two minutes
- Stopping or slowing of breathing during the fainting episode.

WHAT IS A FIT?

A fit, seizure or convulsion is an episode characterised by abnormal movements or feelings, odd behaviour and (most of the time but not always) an altered level of consciousness.

Just because a child has a fit does not mean they have epilepsy. Epilepsy affects just five in 1000 children, and of these only 10 per cent have a serious disorder.

There are several possible underlying causes of seizures in childhood, such as a high temperature (resulting in febrile convulsion), infection of the brain or nervous system, head injury, poisoning, or another systemic disease such as diabetes.

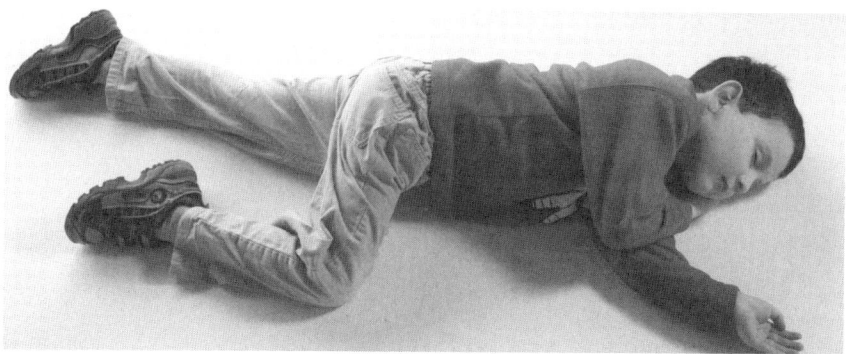

A child in the recovery position. The unconscious child should be placed on the side, with the mouth facing slightly downwards so that any fluids may drain out, and the arms and legs arranged to stabilise the body.

If the seizures are recurrent, there is no fever and no underlying cause is found, then the child may have some form of epilepsy but this requires specialised tests to diagnose correctly.

INITIAL TREATMENT

Whatever the cause of the seizure, the initial management is the same and is aimed at minimising the potentially harmful effects that could result from the seizure.

The priority is to follow the principles of basic life support (see Chapter 24: Basic life support), ensuring that the airway is clear and monitoring the child's breathing and circulation. If the airway is clear and the breathing and pulse are normal, they should be placed in the recovery position, away from any potential hazards that may cause additional injury.

See Chapter 23: The SAFE approach: call for an ambulance (000 in Australia, 111 in New Zealand).

If there is no evidence of breathing or no palpable pulse, basic life support should be started. Children who are known to be epileptic may have medication for seizures that can be given rectally; this should be done by the child's carer who has been instructed in its use.

PREVENTING COMPLICATIONS

The majority of seizures last only a short period – seconds to a few minutes – and need no intervention or treatment. Occasionally, though, the seizure may result in some long-term problems or complications. Simple first aid and quickly seeking expert medical help can reduce the chances of these happening.

It is vital that the airway does not become blocked. During a seizure, control of the muscles around the mouth and throat is lost, and the soft tissues of the mouth can fall back against the throat and obstruct the airway. This can lead to loss of oxygen to the brain and long-term brain injury. The airway should be kept open during a seizure with the jaw thrust (see page 255).

Damage to the brain tissue may occur if the seizure is prolonged. If the seizure does last longer than a couple of minutes, call an ambulance immediately. Paramedics and doctors in the emergency department can stop any further seizures with drugs.

Breathing problems may occur, especially if the body becomes tense and rigid before the shaking begins. In this part of a seizure, children do not breathe and may become cyanosed (blue) because of the lack of oxygen in the blood. It is very rare, however, for them to need assistance with breathing because breathing returns when this brief stage of the seizure ends as long as the airway is open.

Likewise, it is extremely rare for children to need assistance with circulation (CPR or cardiac massage, see page 261) unless the underlying disease process itself affects the heart. The heart rate is increased when a seizure occurs, but it comes back to normal at the end of the episode.

However unlikely these problems are, assessing and treating the complication ensures you never miss them.

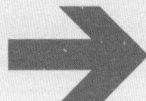

DANGER SIGNS
- Seizures lasting more than two minutes
- Seizures associated with a fever (see opposite)
- Children who look blue (try to open the airway).

INFECTIONS OF THE BRAIN AND SPINAL CORD

Infection of the lining of the brain and spinal cord, the meninges, causes the disease known as meningitis. Meningitis may be caused by a variety of organisms, but bacterial meningitis is the most severe.

Other infections that may affect the brain are encephalitis, an infection of the substance of the brain itself, or an abscess, which is a localised collection of pus that may occur anywhere in the body including the brain. These conditions can affect the child in similar ways and for that reason they will be discussed together.

Meningitis

Bacterial meningitis mainly affects children, with over 80 per cent of all affected patients in Australia and New Zealand being under 16 years old. Awareness and early recognition of the symptoms and signs are the keys to treatment and prevention of serious consequences. The early symptoms are, unfortunately, non-specific (that is, general), especially in infants.

A child with meningitis may be drowsy, or infants floppy, and less responsive than usual. Sometimes the child may have a fit, in which they become unconscious and all their limbs start to shake.

A classic sign of meningitis is a rash. This rash is specific in appearance, being red to purple in colour, occurs in small patches the size of a pinhead or slightly larger and does not turn white when pressed (for example, when a glass is pressed to the skin). This extremely severe problem is called meningococcal septicaemia, and represents the rapid spread of a meningitis bacteria into the blood stream and around the body.

Take action the moment you recognise this disease, as it can lead to rapid collapse, shock and death. If caught early, it can be very effectively treated. If meningitis is suspected, call for an emergency ambulance immediately – 000 in Australia, 111 in New Zealand. The child needs to be taken to the nearest hospital urgently.

TREATMENT

The treatment of infections of the brain involves high doses of antibiotics administered intravenously to reduce the severity of the

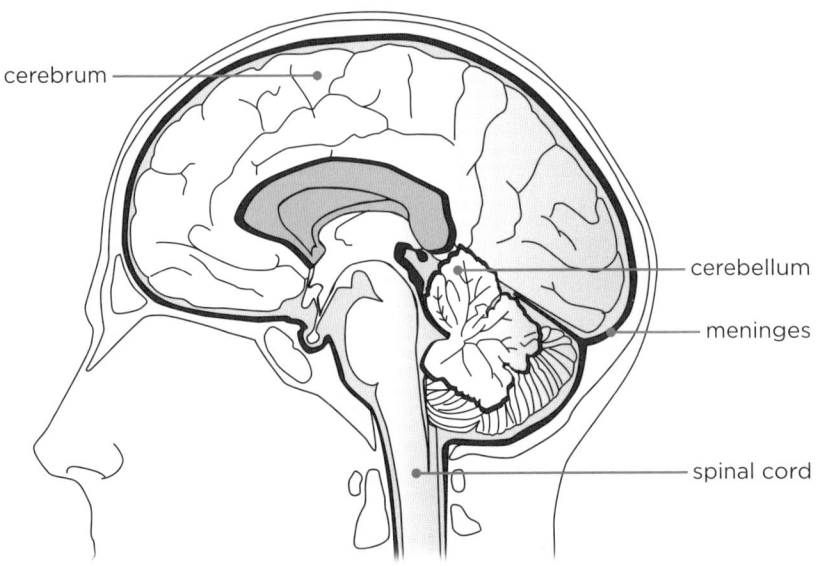

When the meninges – a system of protective membranes that line the brain and the spinal cord – become infected, they become inflamed and cause a number of non-specific symptoms. Meningococcal disease can lead to rapid collapse, shock and death.

illness. Most ambulance services in Australia and New Zealand are able to give urgent antibiotics against meningococcal or other septic shock diseases, and will urgently transport a child with these problems to an emergency department.

FEBRILE CONVULSIONS

If a child is running a high temperature for whatever cause (for example, an ear infection or tonsillitis), they are at risk of having a seizure, or febrile convulsion. These occur in about 3 per cent of children under six years and are commonest between the ages of one and two.

Febrile convulsions are more likely if other family members have a history of similar fits. They usually occur within hours of the onset of fever as the temperature is increasing and are short, lasting only a couple of minutes. Occasionally they recur in the next 24 hours.

SYMPTOMS OF MENINGITIS

Young children

- poor feeding
- lethargy
- fever
- vomiting
- irritability
- drowsiness
- hot in the torso and cold in the limbs
- pale blotchy complexion.

Older children

- headache
- fever – shivering, sweating
- muscle aches
- stiff neck
- photophobia – an aversion to light
- drowsiness
- vomiting
- fitting.

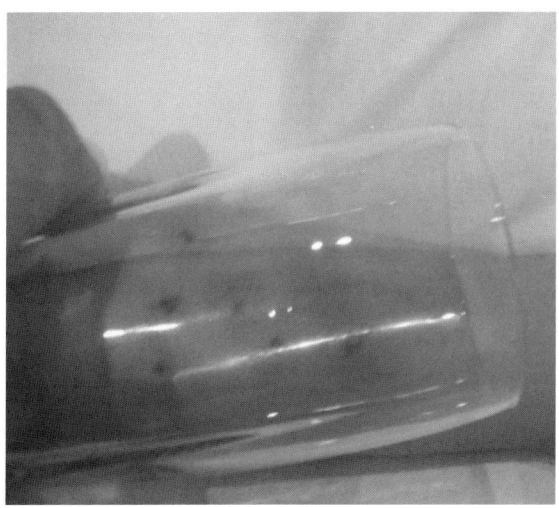

The glass test. The typical rash associated with meningococcal disease does not fade or blanch when pressed with a glass. It is red to purple, and occurs in small patches the size of a pinhead or smaller.

About one-third of children who have a febrile convulsion have another one during their childhood. There is no increased risk of intellectual or growth problems in children with febrile convulsions than in other children of the same age. A small percentage of children with febrile convulsions go on to develop adult epilepsy, but it is not possible to predict who will be affected.

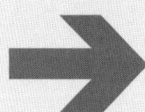

DANGER SIGNS
If your child has a fit coupled with:

- poor feeding
- lethargy
- fever
- irritability
- drowsiness
- high fever
- hot in the torso, cold in the limbs
- any rash

call an ambulance immediately – 000 in Australia, 111 in New Zealand.

TREATMENT

If your child suffers a febrile convulsion, they should be taken to a hospital to be assessed immediately.

Treating the fever – by reducing the temperature – has not been shown to lessen the chances of a further seizure but will still make your child feel better. Reduce their temperature by removing clothing and cooling the environment. Paracetamol or ibuprofen, which specifically reduce fever, should be given (see also Chapter 6: Fevers).

Epilepsy

Epilepsy is a condition of the brain that causes episodic electrical impulses leading to a fit (seizure). There is no obvious cause for most cases of epilepsy, but children can become epileptic after a head injury or meningitis and epilepsy can sometimes run in families. The fits caused by epilepsy can take various forms – usually jerking or twitching of arms and legs, but sometimes only one side of the body is affected, or an absence seizure can occur.

Absence seizure is a form of epilepsy that typically affects the 4-to-12 year age group. It typically causes a spell of 'absence', in which the child loses awareness of the surroundings, appearing vacant. There may be fluttering of the eyes, but usually they will not lose consciousness. Attacks generally only last a couple of minutes and as a rule do not result in any immediate harm. The prognosis is normally good, with 95 per cent of children becoming free of seizures by adolescence.

TREATMENT

The diagnosis of epilepsy can only be made by a paediatrician or a paediatric neurologist. The treatment is usually with medications that stop the brain from firing off abnormal electrical impulses. If your child is on these medications it is important that they are not stopped suddenly as this may predispose them to having a fit.

Parents and carers of children with epilepsy must learn how to recognise when a child is having a fit and the first aid that they may need to administer.

HEAD INJURY

Seizures that occur following a head injury are not uncommon in childhood. They should always be taken seriously because they may herald damage to the structures inside the head, including the brain. For this reason, any child who has a seizure following a head injury should be assessed by a doctor, so that further investigations and treatment can be arranged as necessary.

TREATMENT

All children suffering any type of head injury should be assessed and treated, checking their airways, breathing and circulation, as described in Chapter 24: Basic life support.

DIABETES-RELATED FITS

Diabetes is a condition that affects the body's ability to deal with sugar. It results in a lack of insulin, which is a naturally occurring hormone that helps the body to store and use the sugars in our food. Diabetes can result in abnormal blood sugar levels, which may be either too high or too low, and these can trigger a seizure. Seizures resulting from low blood sugar are referred to as 'hypos' by diabetics.

TREATMENT

If a child is known to be diabetic and suffers a convulsion the assessment of their airways, breathing and circulation is required, as with all fits, along with urgent treatment of the potential low blood sugars – call an ambulance. These seizures are often associated with a preceding decreased level of consciousness, shaking and a clammy feel to the skin.

These symptoms of a 'hypo' should be treated by the immediate ingestion of sugars; this can be in the form of sugar drinks, sweets or gel (but do not put anything in the mouth of an unconscious patient). This can help to prevent a seizure from occurring.

DRUGS AND ALCOHOL

An increasing problem among older children and teenagers is the use of drugs and alcohol, which are now a common cause of seizures in this age group. The use of ecstasy, for example, is on the increase and it is responsible for some hospital admissions for seizures and other related conditions. Infants and younger children can unwittingly take these drugs, which may look innocent to a child.

Children suffering seizures secondary to poisoning, especially of prescription drugs or household poisons, represent a group at high risk of serious illness and death.

Again, all children should have airways, breathing and circulation assessed and an emergency ambulance should be called. Any evidence of drug use should mean a visit to the hospital, because specific treatment may be required, depending on the type of drug that has been taken.

At the hospital

Most frequently, by the time the child arrives at the hospital, a seizure will be over and they will be in a state referred to as 'post-ictal' or post-seizure by the time they see a medical practitioner. Often this means they are very drowsy, with various levels of confusion or decreased level of consciousness. When you arrive at the emergency department your child will be assessed and triaged depending on the severity of the illness. If they look very unwell or have not fully regained consciousness they will be assessed as a priority and seen quickly. If they look well and are not distressed they may have to wait a while until more urgent cases are dealt with.

Always attempt to give a clear and concise history (see pages 55, 268) to the medical personnel. It will help them diagnose the problem and judge the severity of the illness. The paramedics or hospital teams will take over airway and breathing management and perform a quick primary assessment. They will assess oxygenation with a small device placed on the finger and will do a quick neurological examination. Very early in the assessment, the blood sugar will be tested – this is a very important part of the immediate examination because it may show a rapidly reversible cause of the seizure and prevent further acute problems.

Once the child's stability is assured a more complete exam will be performed, including temperature measurement. If a diagnosis of febrile convulsion is made, the medical staff will hopefully find an explanation for this. Paracetamol or ibuprofen will be given to reduce the fever. Children probably will have already lost some temperature with exposure during the initial examination so it is not uncommon for temperatures to normalise in an emergency department. The amount of clothes left on is determined by the child's comfort and environment.

A clinical examination, especially when repeated over a few hours, remains the best tool for gauging if there is a serious problem. Investigations – such as urine tests (to rule out urinary tract infections), blood tests (to look at the salts and infective markers in the blood), chest x-ray or CT scan of the head – may be necessary.

The tests performed are dependent on the presenting history and state of the child. Blood tests may be done where there is suspicion of a metabolic disorder or severe illness, and very rarely a CT scan will be performed. Usually this is reserved for post-traumatic seizures or where the level of consciousness remains altered with no clear cause. The CT scan delivers a substantial radiation dose, and although it must be performed when necessary, careful thought should come first as well as discussion between doctors and parents or carers.

After the examination and investigations, the medical staff will decide if your child will need to be admitted to the hospital for further assessment. When they can go home will depend on their displaying a normal level of consciousness and taking oral food or fluids, thereby demonstrating no residual or underlying problems. A follow-up consultation with your GP for simple febrile convulsions may be advised, and anything else should usually be with a paediatrician or paediatric neurologist depending on where you live and what services are available locally.

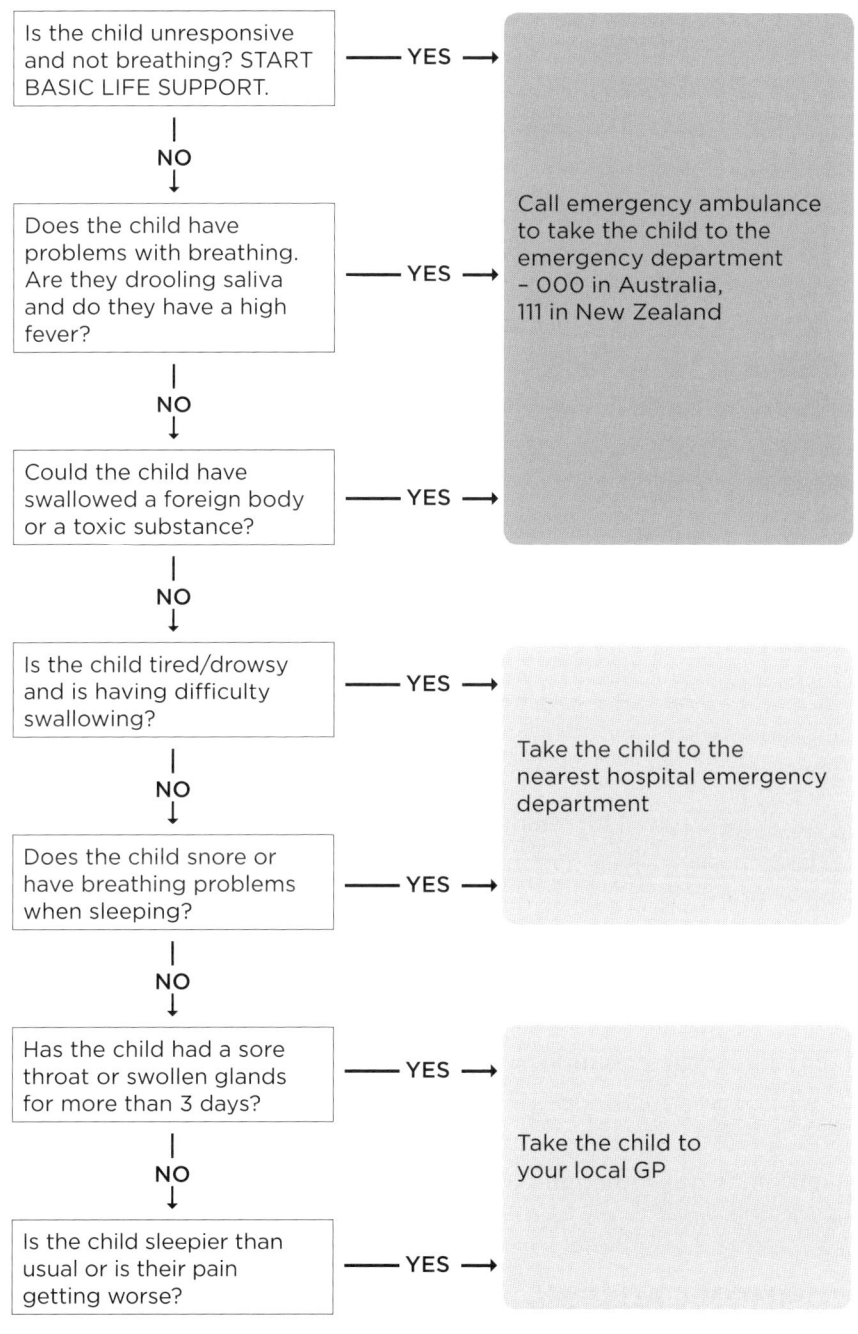

Is the child unresponsive and not breathing? START BASIC LIFE SUPPORT. —— YES →

NO ↓

Does the child have problems with breathing. Are they drooling saliva and do they have a high fever? —— YES →

NO ↓

Could the child have swallowed a foreign body or a toxic substance? —— YES →

Call emergency ambulance to take the child to the emergency department – 000 in Australia, 111 in New Zealand

NO ↓

Is the child tired/drowsy and is having difficulty swallowing? —— YES →

NO ↓

Does the child snore or have breathing problems when sleeping? —— YES →

Take the child to the nearest hospital emergency department

NO ↓

Has the child had a sore throat or swollen glands for more than 3 days? —— YES →

NO ↓

Is the child sleepier than usual or is their pain getting worse? —— YES →

Take the child to your local GP

11

Headaches

It is not uncommon for children to have headaches. Older children, and teenagers especially, report having several headaches a year. Most are minor. But there are some danger signs for more serious headaches.

A headache can be a frightening experience, even though the vast majority are benign in nature. They can be frustrating for the child, parents and the doctors trying to find out what has caused them. By far the commonest type of childhood headaches are tension headaches and migraines.

A lot of headaches, including migraines, have 'triggers' that start them off. It can sometimes be difficult to find a cause for a headache because physical, emotional or psychological factors can be involved.

COMMON CAUSES

The most important factor with childhood headaches is to exclude rare but serious causes. There are symptoms and signs that will alert you to the more worrying headaches.

Most headaches occur infrequently and are not severe (or very painful) in nature. A headache may be a sign of another illness. It may be associated with fever, infections of the throat or ear, or congestion of the nose or sinuses. The commonest types are: tension or stress (psychogenic), migraine and headaches occurring after head trauma.

A tension headache usually feels like a tight band around the head, sometimes with an ache in the neck and shoulder muscles as well. It is caused by contraction or spasm of the muscles in the head and neck. Many things can lead to this, such as sitting in the same position for too long (as when playing computer games), and emotional problems such as stress (at home or at school) and feeling anxious or depressed. Tension headaches caused by emotional problems (known as stress or psychogenic headaches) are often associated with physical problems such as weight loss, sleeping problems and loss of appetite.

After trauma to the head or a head injury it is common to have a headache (like having pain or an ache in your ankle after twisting it). But constant or severe headaches, especially if they are associated with increasing drowsiness or loss of consciousness, vomiting or problems with hearing or seeing, may indicate damage to the brain. If your child has any of these symptoms, you should take them to the nearest emergency department. If you are very worried about them, call an ambulance.

Serious headaches

Causes of serious headaches in children include:

- meningitis
- encephalitis
- brain tumour
- severe headache after a head injury
- intracranial haemorrhage.

Meningitis and encephalitis are infections of the linings of the brain and of the brain tissue respectively (see page 129).

The first signs of a brain tumour, which are rare in children, can be chronic recurrent headaches. Children with brain tumours usually have other worrying symptoms as well as headaches – for example, speech difficulties, episodes of confusion, visual difficulties, weight loss, fits, vomiting and drowsiness. Headaches associated with tumours are often worse in the mornings. If your child has headaches associated with any of these symptoms, you should take them to a doctor to get checked out as a matter of urgency.

TREATMENT

For mild headaches that do not occur too often, paracetamol or ibuprofen may be taken to ease the pain. If your child has more severe headaches take them to your GP, who can prescribe stronger painkillers and investigate the underlying causes. It is important to rule out sinister causes in headaches of increasing severity and/or frequency. Any obvious triggers that have caused the headaches should be avoided.

MIGRAINES

Migraines are recurrent and can affect children in a wide variety of ways. The headaches can range from fairly mild to very severe, and they can come with a frequency from less than one a year to more than one a week. Migraines are not serious or life threatening, but they can be debilitating and may last for several hours.

Sometimes migraines run in families, and sometimes it is possible to pinpoint a trigger that causes the headache (common triggers are chocolate, cheese, caffeine, alcohol and being tired or dehydrated). The pain that migraines cause varies from child to child. They tend to be throbbing in nature and often affect one side of the head only. They are commonly associated with nausea and vomiting. Some children also complain of visual disturbances (such as seeing flashing lights).

Migraine is not a diagnosis that doctors should make without considering – and eliminating – all other potential causes.

TREATMENT

There is no general cure or prevention for migraine headaches, so it is advisable to avoid known triggers, if any can be found. At the onset of a migraine painkillers should be given. There are some medicines that are especially good at treating a migraine – these are usually only prescribed to children with very regular or very severe migraines. Children who suffer severe recurrent migraines may also be prescribed medications that may prevent the headache.

At the doctor's

If your child looks very unwell or has a severe headache with vomiting, they will be made a priority and seen quickly. If they look well and are not distressed, they may have to wait a while before being seen.

Your child will be examined and some observations will be performed (usually pulse and respiratory rate, and oxygen levels – a small probe on their finger or foot). A clinical examination remains the best tool for gauging if there is a serious problem.

Investigations may include urine tests (to rule out urinary tract infections), blood tests (to look at the salts and infective markers in the blood), chest x-ray or a CT scan of the head. After the examination and investigations the medical staff will decide if your child can go home or will need to be admitted to the hospital for further assessment.

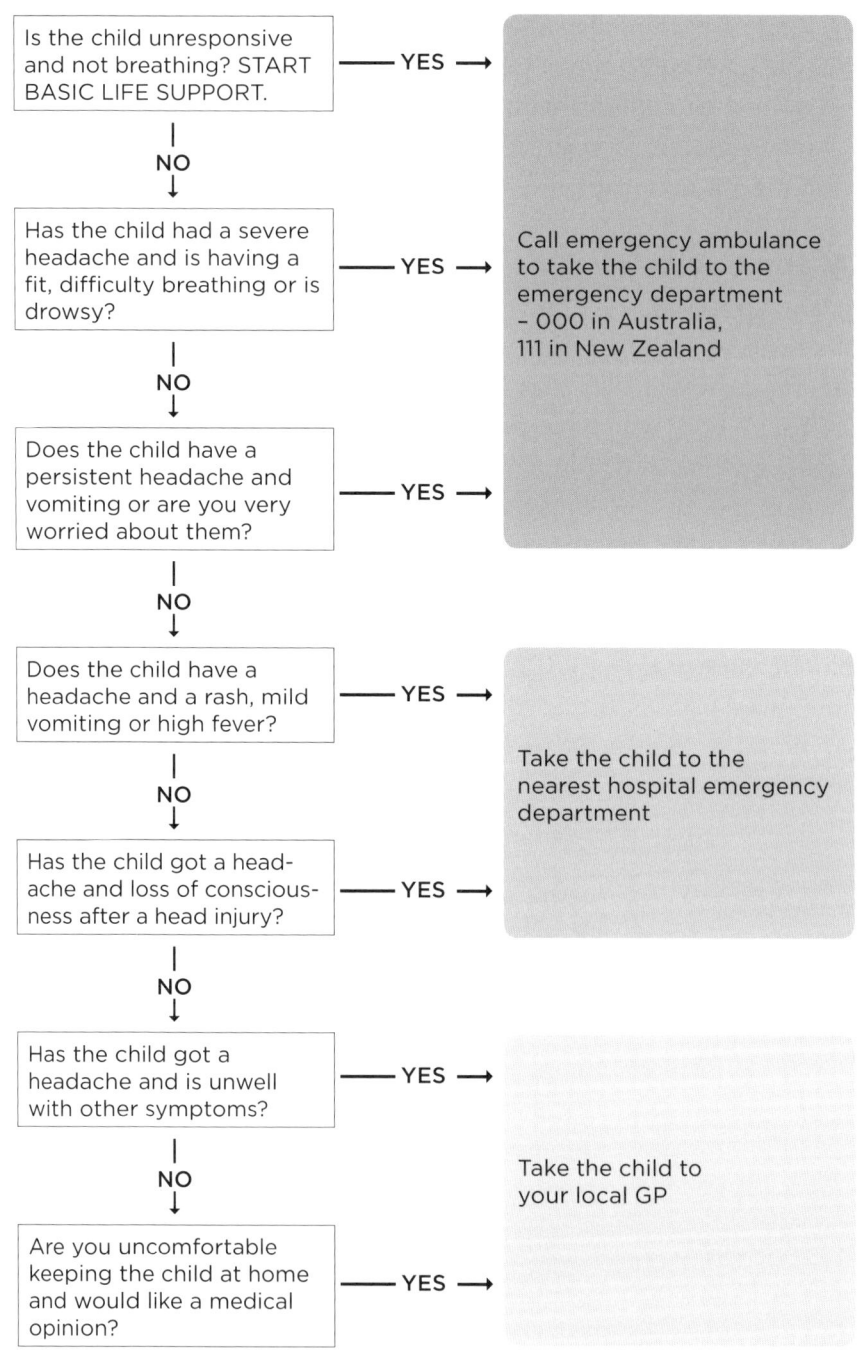

Is the child unresponsive and not breathing? START BASIC LIFE SUPPORT. —— YES →

NO ↓

Has the child had a severe headache and is having a fit, difficulty breathing or is drowsy? —— YES →

NO ↓

Does the child have a persistent headache and vomiting or are you very worried about them? —— YES →

Call emergency ambulance to take the child to the emergency department – 000 in Australia, 111 in New Zealand

NO ↓

Does the child have a headache and a rash, mild vomiting or high fever? —— YES →

NO ↓

Has the child got a head-ache and loss of conscious-ness after a head injury? —— YES →

Take the child to the nearest hospital emergency department

NO ↓

Has the child got a headache and is unwell with other symptoms? —— YES →

NO ↓

Take the child to your local GP

Are you uncomfortable keeping the child at home and would like a medical opinion? —— YES →

12

RASHES AND SKIN CONDITIONS

Finding a rash on your child can be worrying, knowing that the first sign of meningitis can be a rash. However, rashes in childhood are very common and meningitis is very rare.

There are many causes of these rashes. Unlike adults, children frequently get rashes with viral infections, and other typical childhood diseases also cause rashes. They may feel hot and/or cause itchiness, which can be very uncomfortable.

Nevertheless, there are some rare instances of serious causes of rashes in children – in particular, you need to beware of meningitis and anaphylactic reactions.

WHAT IS A RASH?

A rash is a reaction in the skin, and because children's skin is more sensitive than adult's, rashes tend to more common in childhood.

The reaction in skin that causes a rash is usually due to an infection (viral or bacterial), an allergy or a medicine.

COMMON TYPES AND CAUSES OF CHILDHOOD RASHES

Viral
- general viral rash
- chicken pox
- measles
- hand, foot and mouth disease.

Bacterial
- impetigo
- scarlet fever (scarletina).

Allergic
- allergy – urticaria
- drug or medicine related
- erythema multiforme.

Other
- eczema
- psoriasis.

RASHES FROM VIRAL INFECTION

With viral illnesses – such as upper respiratory tract infections (see Chapter 5: Infections), sore throats (see Chapter 15: Sore throats and swollen glands), ear infections (see Chapter 14: Earaches and hearing problems) and gastroenteritis (see Chapter 9: Vomiting and diarrhoea) – a child might develop a rash, which is simply a reaction in the skin due to the virus circulating in the blood.

These generalised viral rashes can vary in appearance but are usually pink or pale red, flat, patchy and not itchy. They will resolve over the course of a few days as your child recovers from the viral illness. If your child has a fever and a rash and if you are not sure of the cause you should take them to see your GP.

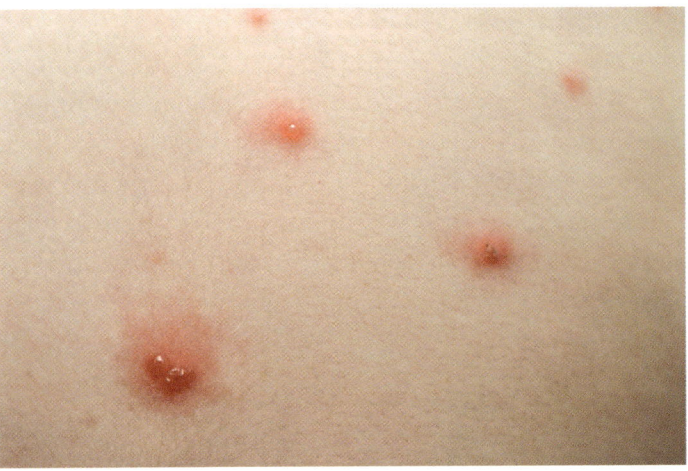

A typical chicken pox rash.

Chicken pox

Chicken pox is caused by the varicella virus – 'varicella' is another name for chicken pox. Like most viral infections it causes a fever, a rash and other non-specific symptoms (such as tiredness, headache, sore throat). The chicken pox rash is fairly distinctive – individual pimples which become blisters that burst, forming a crust. The rash usually starts on the chest or back and then spreads to the face and to the rest of the body, and is extremely itchy. It is also possible for the varicella virus to affect the brain, as in encephalitis (see page 129), or the lungs, causing pneumonia (see page 89).

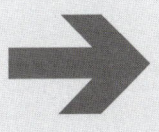

DANGER SIGNS
If your child has chicken pox and becomes very unwell, take them to the nearest emergency department.

TREATMENT

Being a virus, varicella cannot be treated with antibiotics. However, the itchiness from the rash can be controlled with lotions such as calamine, and the fever and other viral symptoms may be treated with paracetamol or ibuprofen. Chicken pox is contagious – you should keep your child away from other children until the blistered parts of the rash have dried up. Vaccination is now part of the normal immunisation schedule, starting at 18 months of age (see page 77).

In rare cases, there may be serious complications with chicken pox, when the blisters can become infected with staphylococcal or streptococcal bacteria (see Impetigo, opposite) and need treatment with antibiotics.

Measles

Measles is also caused by a viral infection (paramyxovirus). Measles has become very rare since immunisation became available for children in Australia and New Zealand as part of the MMR vaccine (see pages 77, 286). However, the disease is responsible for the deaths of many children in the world each year, especially in third world countries where vaccination programs are not available. There is no evidence to support suggestions that the MMR vaccine may lead to increased incidences of autism in children. There is irrefutable evidence that measles kills many children worldwide each year.

Children with measles start to show mild symptoms – a runny nose, red eyes – and feel generally unwell. The rash comes out after

The measles rash (left) and hand, foot and mouth disease (right) with blisters on the soles of the feet.

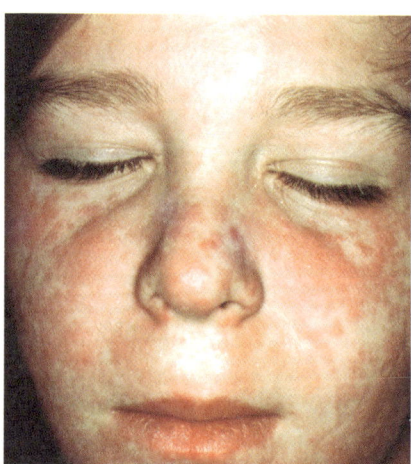
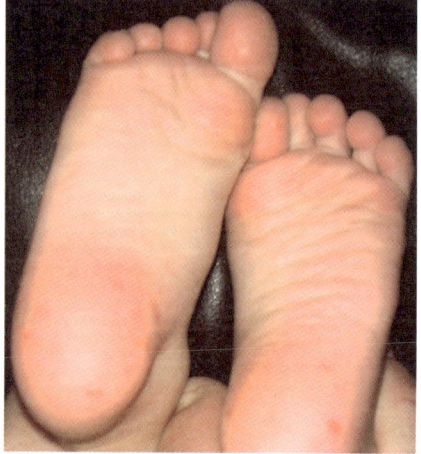

a few days – typically, dark purple or brown in colour. It starts on the face, spreads down to the chest and then to the rest of the body.

As with chicken pox infection, the measles virus can lead to some very serious complications, including encephalitis, pneumonia, ear infections and diarrhoea. There is also a very rare but always fatal condition known as SSPE (subacute sclerosing panencephalitis), which does not occur until a couple of years after the measles illness.

TREATMENT
As with all viral infections, there is no specific treatment, but you can make your child feel more comfortable with paracetamol or ibuprofen.

Hand, foot and mouth disease
This is caused by a family of viruses called coxsackie viruses. Children typically have a generalised viral rash and a fever. They will also have painful blisters on the palms of the hands, soles of the feet and the inside of the lips and on the tongue. Other than the similar name, there is no link between this disease and the foot and mouth disease suffered by cattle and other livestock.

TREATMENT
As with all viral infections, there is no specific treatment, but you can make your child feel more comfortable with paracetamol or ibuprofen.

RASHES FROM BACTERIAL INFECTION
Rashes due to bacterial infections can also take on many different forms. In general, any rash that has a yellow discharge, pus or a golden-coloured crust is probably due to a bacterial infection. Other examples are given below.

Impetigo
Impetigo is caused when the skin is infected by a bacteria called staphylococcus or streptococcus. Most of us carry these bacteria on our skin normally (in fact, our skin naturally has millions of bacteria),

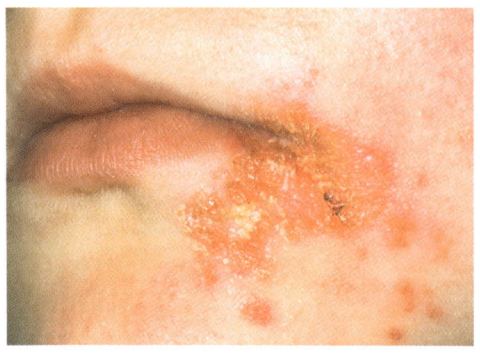

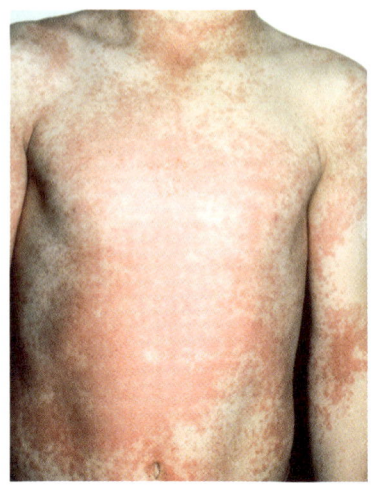

The impetigo rash (above) usually appears on the face.
The scarlet fever rash (right).

but occasionally when a break develops in the skin these bacteria can lead to an infection. Impetigo causes collections of infected blisters, typically with a golden-coloured crust. These tend to occur in groups, mostly on the face, especially around the mouth and nose, and can easily be spread to other parts of the body by touch. Impetigo is contagious, so you will need to keep your child away from other children until the rash has dried up.

TREATMENT
Impetigo is treated with antibiotics which are either administered topically (an ointment or cream applied to the skin) or orally (tablets or medicine).

Scarlet fever

Scarlet fever is an infection caused by streptococcus bacteria which results in a sore throat, fever, swollen red tongue and a rash. It is also known as scarletina (see Chapter 15: Sore throats and swollen glands). The rash is pale pink and looks a bit like sunburn but can feel quite rough to the touch (like sandpaper).

TREATMENT
If you think your child has scarlet fever you should take them to your GP or paediatrician. It is treated with a course of penicillin.

SKIN RASHES DUE TO ALLERGY

These are usually easy to diagnose. There is often a history of allergy, or the substance that has caused a local reaction can be determined. Allergic rashes (or urticaria) are usually red, raised, patchy and itchy.

TREATMENT

The treatment for these rashes is to identify and avoid the cause, and to use oral or topical antihistamines to control the itch. Be watchful for other symptoms in a child with an allergic rash to make sure they don't have an anaphylactic reaction (see page 153).

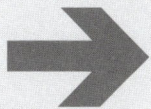

DANGER SIGNS

If your child has an allergic rash with an airway, breathing or circulation problem, you need to take them to the nearest emergency department immediately or call for an ambulance – 000 in Australia, 111 in New Zealand.

DRUG- OR MEDICINE-RELATED RASHES

Erythema multiforme is a skin reaction that occurs after the body is exposed either to an infection or a drug/medicine. It is thought to be an overreaction by the immune system and is more common in

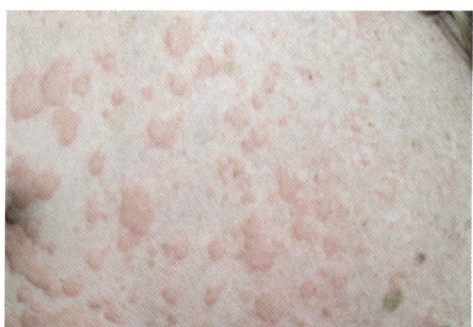
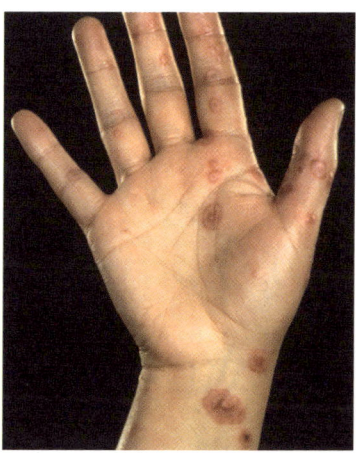

An allergy rash (above) is raised and itchy. The skin rash of erythema multiforme (right).

children than in adults, possibly because a child's immune system is still maturing. Usually it shows up as isolated or discrete patches on the skin that look pink or red with a pale centre, known as target lesions. Erythema multiforme can vary from a mild reaction (with a self-limiting skin rash) to a severe and life-threatening condition, known as Stevens-Johnson syndrome, when the rash on the mouth, anus and genitals is so severe the skin can peel off.

TREATMENT

If you think your child has any of these, take them to your GP.

OTHER RASHES

The skin conditions described above are all temporary – they will go away either on their own or with specific treatment and very rarely recur. There are some skin conditions that are chronic (long-term) in nature. The most common are eczema and psoriasis.

Eczema

This is also known as dermatitis and it produces red, itchy and dry skin. It is associated with asthma and allergies and can run in families.

TREATMENT

The main treatment is to keep the skin moisturised. Your GP or pharmacist will be able to give you advice about how to best achieve this, and some things to do to prevent the eczema from worsening

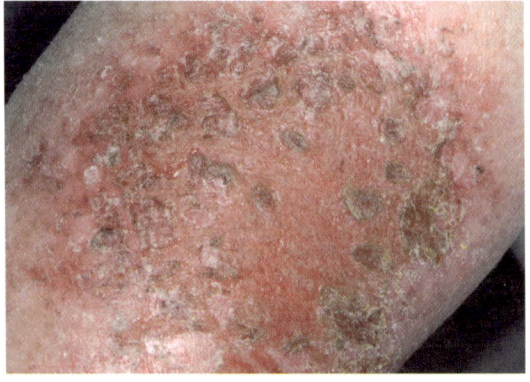

A flare up of eczema: red, itchy and dry skin.

– for example, bathing with oil added to the bathwater, applying a good neutral skin cream twice a day, and seeking medical attention if the affected skin starts to look red and angry. Sometimes for 'active' eczema your child will need a mild steroid cream to be prescribed.

Psoriasis

Psoriasis also produces a red, dry, scaly and itchy rash. It is more common on the elbows and knees. It is sometimes difficult to tell the difference between eczema and psoriasis – see your doctor for advice.

TREATMENT

Like eczema, this needs to be treated by keeping the skin moist.

SERIOUS SKIN CONDITIONS

Serious causes of a rash in a child can result from meningitis, erythema multiforme and anaphylactic reaction.

Meningitis often starts as a rash in an otherwise well child, who then deteriorates rapidly to become severely unwell (see page 129). The meningitis rash is specific in appearance, being red to purple in

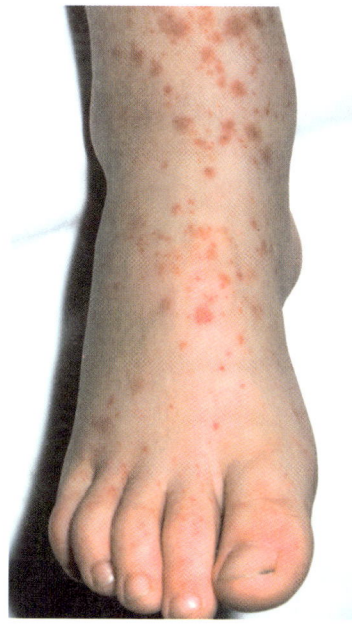

The word 'purpura' means purple – the purpura rash associated with meningitis is red to purple in colour and occurs in small clusters.

colour in small patches the size of a pinhead or slightly larger, and does not turn white when pressed (for example, when a glass is being pressed to the skin).

Erythema multiforme can vary from a mild rash in an otherwise well child to a severe rash in a child who is critically unwell. Allergic rashes are common but an anaphylactic reaction, on the other hand, is much less common.

Anaphylactic reaction

In this condition not just the skin but other body systems are affected by the allergic reaction. Anaphylaxis quickly becomes life threatening. A combination of symptoms involving the airway (swollen lips, tongue and throat), breathing (wheezing and difficult breathing) and circulation (fast pulse and low blood pressure) are seen. Apart from these problems, other body systems can be affected: the child may have abdominal pain, vomiting or diarrhoea, may feel dizzy or simply 'feel strange'. The speed of the onset and change of these symptoms are specific for allergic reactions.

TREATMENT

Immediate treatment with a drug called adrenaline is needed. Antihistamines, which are frequently used for milder allergies, have little effect in anaphylaxis and their use may delay the treatment that definitely works.

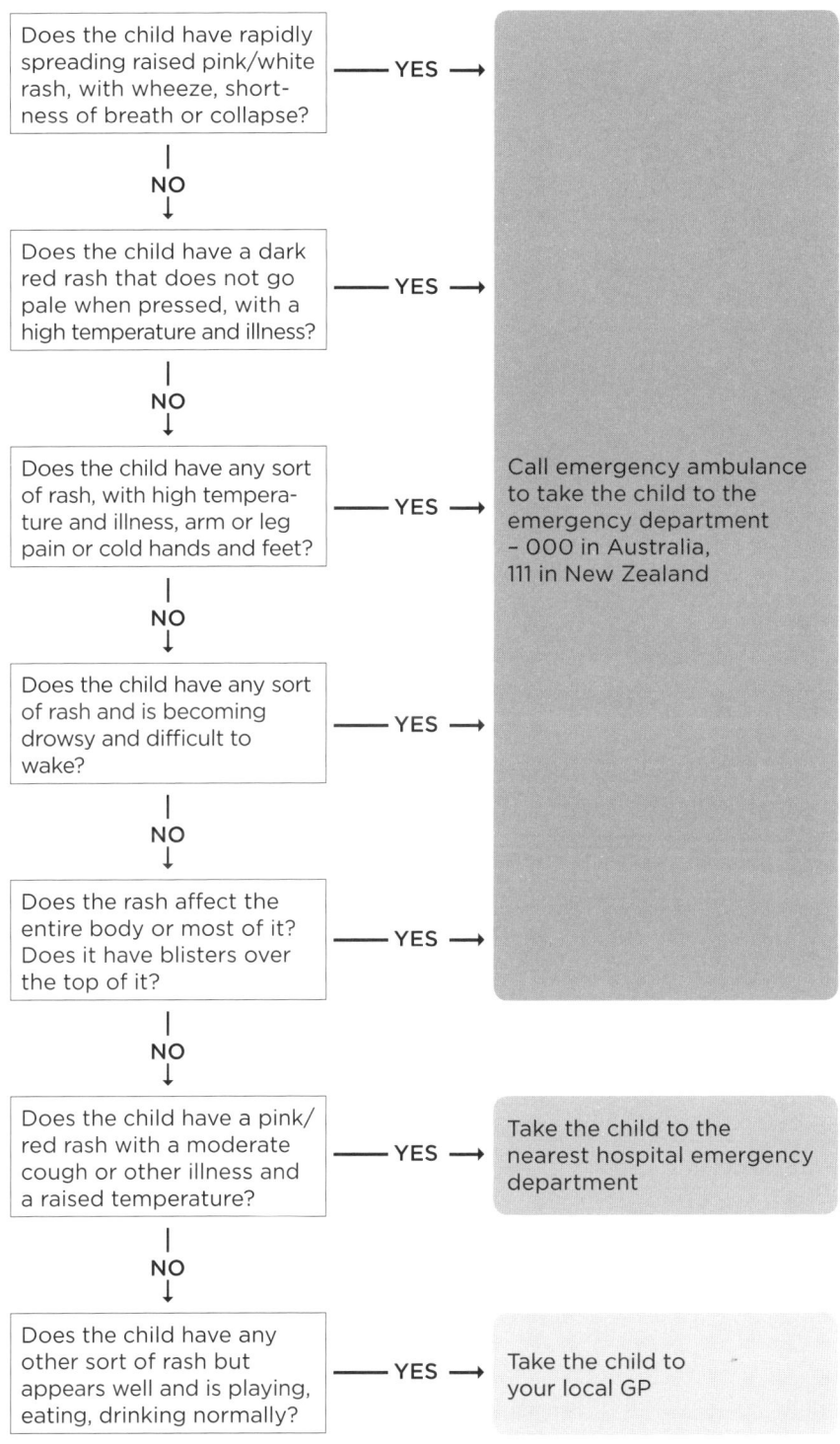

Does the child have rapidly spreading raised pink/white rash, with wheeze, shortness of breath or collapse? —— YES →

NO ↓

Does the child have a dark red rash that does not go pale when pressed, with a high temperature and illness? —— YES →

NO ↓

Does the child have any sort of rash, with high temperature and illness, arm or leg pain or cold hands and feet? —— YES →

NO ↓

Does the child have any sort of rash and is becoming drowsy and difficult to wake? —— YES →

NO ↓

Does the rash affect the entire body or most of it? Does it have blisters over the top of it? —— YES →

NO ↓

Call emergency ambulance to take the child to the emergency department – 000 in Australia, 111 in New Zealand

Does the child have a pink/red rash with a moderate cough or other illness and a raised temperature? —— YES → Take the child to the nearest hospital emergency department

NO ↓

Does the child have any other sort of rash but appears well and is playing, eating, drinking normally? —— YES → Take the child to your local GP

13

EYE
PROBLEMS

This chapter concentrates on the acute problems that can affect children's eyes, how to recognise them and what you need to do about them. It does not aim to cover the more long-term eye problems such as eyesight limitation, blindness, squint or cataracts.

ANATOMY OF AN EYE

It is important to have a basic understanding of the anatomy of the eye because this will allow you to see how diseases, infections and injuries to the eye can occur and the symptoms and signs that they will cause.

The eyelids are the protectors of the eye – as well as protecting the eyeball by covering it, you blink to prevent things entering your eye, and the blinking distributes lubricant over the surface of the eye. The front white surface of the eye is the conjunctiva, which forms a covering over the eyeball and loops back on itself inside the eye socket (this is why you can never 'lose' an eyelash or a contact lens

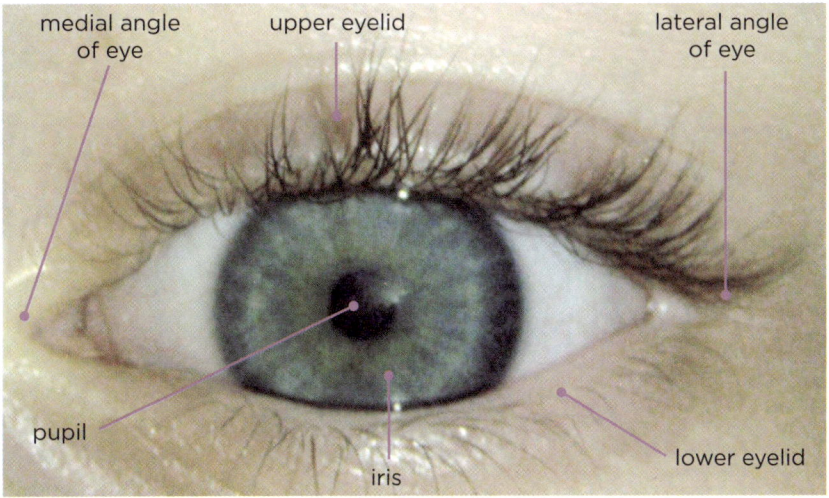

The front part of the outer layer of the eye, the cornea, refracts light. It is transparent, allowing the iris, and its centre, the pupil, to be seen. The retina, the inner layer of the eye, is made up of a series of rod and cone cells that react to light, like the film in a camera.

behind the eye). The iris is the coloured part of the eyeball (blue, green or brown in most people), with the pupil (the black circle) at its centre. Light enters the eye through the pupil and is then directed by the lens (the part that can become cloudy, forming a cataract) onto the back of the eye (or retina).

RED EYE

Probably the most common eye problem in children is red eye. This is when the conjunctiva (the white front surface of the eye) looks pink or red. Often the eye also feels painful, itchy or has some discharge (yellow, green or crusty).

The most common causes of a red eye in children are: bacterial conjunctivitis, viral conjunctivitis, allergy or hay fever, trauma to the eye, and foreign bodies in the eye.

Bacterial conjunctivitis

Bacterial conjunctivitis is probably the main reason children get red eye, and it is characterised by an itchy eye with yellow, green or crusty

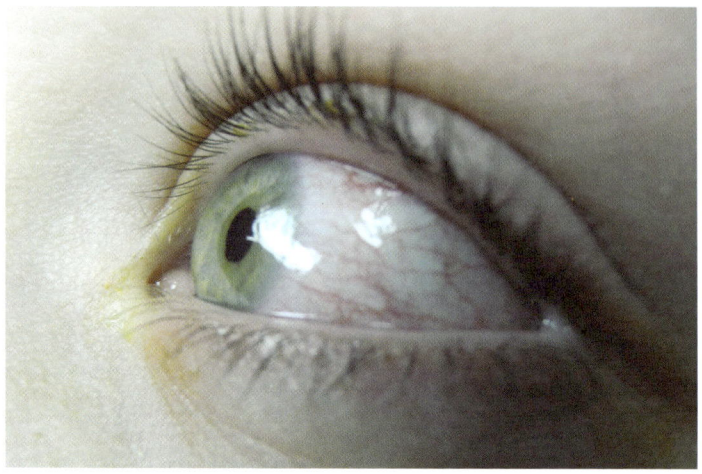

There are many causes of red eye, including conjunctivitis, allergy or hay fever and injury.

discharge that may stick the eyelids and eyelashes together. It usually starts in one eye, with the other quickly becoming involved.

TREATMENT

Gently washing the eye with cotton wool balls soaked in warm water will clear the discharge, but antibiotic drops, ointment or tablets will be needed to clear the infection – you will have to take your child to your GP.

Bacterial conjunctivitis can spread easily to other children so keep your child isolated, which will mean keeping them home instead of going to childcare, school or the playground until they have had at least 24 hours of the antibiotics.

Viral conjunctivitis

Viral conjunctivitis is almost always associated with other symptoms and signs of a viral infection, such as snotty nose, sore throat, cough and fever. This condition usually affects both eyes and will resolve spontaneously without any specific treatment. It is sometimes difficult to tell viral from bacterial conjunctivitis, so your doctor might decide to treat it with antibiotics.

Allergies or fever

Children whose eyes are red due to allergy or hay fever have itchy and very watery eyes. They will also have other symptoms and signs of these conditions, such as a runny nose, sneezing, an itchy cough and usually a history of allergy.

TREATMENT

There are many different eye drops that can help in these circumstances and you should seek advice from your GP or pharmacist.

INFECTIONS AROUND THE EYE

There are two serious infections that occur around the eye: periorbital cellulitis and orbital cellulitis. These infections affect one side of the face only. Periorbital cellulitis means infection of the skin and tissues around the eye; orbital cellulitis is an infection of the eyeball itself.

In periorbital cellulitis the eyelids become red and inflamed, sometimes so swollen that the child finds it difficult to open their eye. But the eye underneath is not affected – it is not red, and their eye will be normal.

Orbital cellulitis is an extremely serious and sight-threatening condition. The eyelids may be affected, as in periorbital cellulitis, but the eyeball is also affected. Your child will have a painful red eye and their vision will be impaired. Moving the eye to look at things may cause pain.

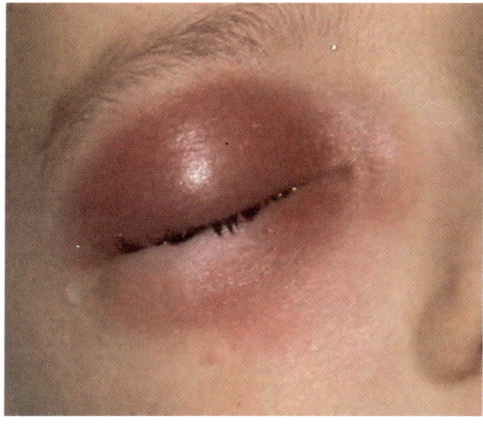

Red, inflamed eyelids are a sign of serious infection and the child should be taken to an emergency department.

TREATMENT

Both of these conditions need assessment and treatment in a hospital, so you should take your child to an emergency department if you suspect them.

Periorbital cellulitis needs to be treated with antibiotics, often strong ones that need to be given intravenously (so your child will have to have a drip).

Orbital cellulitis is an emergency problem and often needs urgent surgery to correct, as well as antibiotics administered via a drip to treat the infection.

EYE INJURIES

Any injury or trauma to the eye or eyelids can potentially affect vision. Cuts to the eyelids can sometimes go through into the eyeball, and small fragments of glass or metal may penetrate the outer protective conjunctiva and also enter the eyeball.

TREATMENT

All of these injuries must be seen by a doctor: your GP, an emergency department or an ophthalmologist. These injuries need to be assessed with specialised equipment to allow the inside of the eye to be examined in detail.

FOREIGN BODIES

Foreign bodies often can penetrate into the front of the eye. The most common examples of these are eyelashes or a piece of sand, dust or dirt. The conjunctiva prevents them from ending up behind the eyeball (see page 154), but they tend to become stuck either on the conjunctiva or underneath the upper eyelid.

Sometimes foreign bodies become dislodged very quickly, but they leave the sensation that something is still there (known as a 'foreign body sensation'), when really there is just a small scratch on the conjunctiva.

TREATMENT

If you think your child has something in their eye you can try to rinse it out with warm tap water. If this is not successful or if you have successfully removed the object but their eye is still painful, you should go to your GP. The eye and under the eyelids can then be properly examined.

Often the foreign body causes a scratch or abrasion to the surface of the eye and antibiotic drops or ointment may be prescribed to prevent the scratch becoming infected.

If your child gets any sort of liquid or chemical in their eye, rinse the eye immediately with copious amounts of warm water. Check what the substance is and seek urgent advice from your GP, emergency department or poisons centre (Poisons Information Centre Australia: 13 11 26; Poisons Information Centre New Zealand: 0800 764 766). If you know the substance is an acid or an alkali (bleach, for example), you should call an ambulance to take your child to hospital – chemical injuries can be potentially blinding.

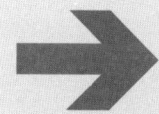

DANGER SIGNS
Red eye
- if associated with either pain or decrease in vision.

Redness around the eye (periorbital cellulitis)
- if associated with pain in the eye and decrease in vision – this is an emergency
- foreign body in the eye that you cannot wash out
- any acid or alkali that enters the eye.

14

EARACHES AND HEARING PROBLEMS

Earaches are fairly common in childhood; they are due mostly to infection with a virus. Some children develop chronic (long-term) ear infections, including glue ear, which may need surgical treatment. Hearing problems due to glue ear or other problems can occur in infancy. About 20 per cent of children under four years of age will experience an ear infection at least once a year. This means that by the age of four it is extremely likely that your child will have suffered at least one ear infection. Most of these infections will last two to three days and clear up on their own.

There are two main areas of the ear that can be infected: the outer ear and the middle ear. The infections cause different symptoms and are treated in different ways. In Australia and New Zealand all babies should have their hearing tested in the first few months of life as part of normal newborn screening. Hearing problems after this time are often noticed by parents or teachers. Concern about hearing in any child should be referred for specialist assessment and hearing testing.

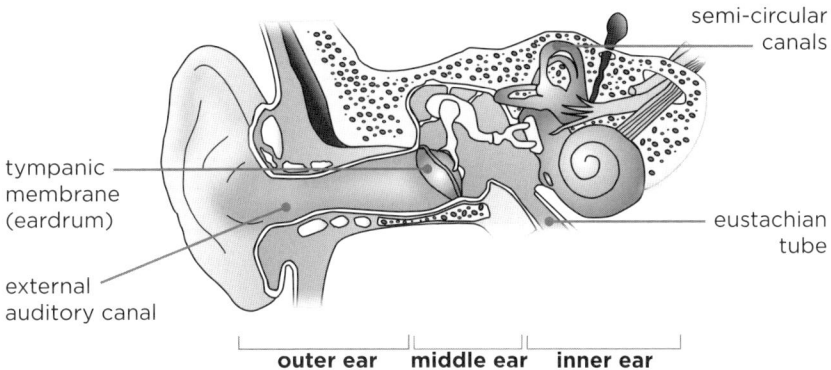

semi-circular canals

tympanic membrane (eardrum)

external auditory canal

eustachian tube

outer ear   middle ear   inner ear

The ear has three layers. Sound waves travel through the ear canal and vibrate against the eardrum, then pass through the middle ear into the shell-shaped cochlea in the inner ear, where they are transmitted to the brain.

EARACHES

By far the most common cause of an earache in a child is an acute ear infection. Painful ears may also be a result of trauma (being hit in the ear or falling onto that side of the head) or caused by a foreign body being put into the ear canal (see Chapter 20: Poisoning and foreign bodies). A child with an ear infection may complain of pain in the ear or may pull at the affected ear. In older babies and infants pulling

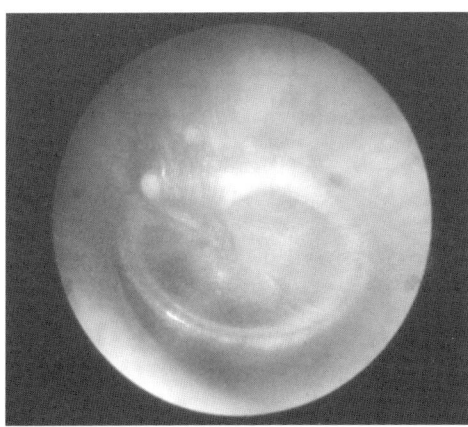

Glue ear is an infection of the middle ear caused by a collection of fluid behind the eardrum.

at the ear is particularly common and may be the only clue that there is an ear infection. An earache may also cause your child to have a fever and to feel unwell.

Serious complications of ear infections, such as the spread of the infection to the lining of the brain (known as meningitis, see page 129) and to the bones around the ear (known as mastoiditis) are very uncommon but very serious. All children who have a fever and pain in the ear should have their ears examined by a doctor.

TREATMENT

The majority of ear infections do not benefit from being treated with antibiotics because – as with most upper respiratory tract infections – they are usually caused by a viral infection. In 50 per cent of ear infections a child will get better within two to three days without any treatment; pain and fever associated with the infection can be alleviated with paracetamol or ibuprofen.

An ear infection associated with a high fever (greater than 38.5°C) that persists for over 48 hours or with vomiting is more likely to benefit from antibiotics because these other symptoms may indicate that it is a bacterial infection.

Middle ear infections

Infections of the middle ear (the part of the ear behind the eardrum) are the most common ear infections in childhood. These infections are called otitis media (meaning 'inflamed middle ear'). They are often related to a viral cold-like illness affecting the upper respiratory passages and, because there is a link between the back of the throat and the middle ear, infection can travel directly between these two areas. Pus may accumulate in the middle ear space and the eardrum can become tense and swollen.

Recurrent ear infections may lead to glue ear, a chronic (long-term) condition in which there is secretion of thick mucus-like fluid into the middle ear. Glue ear may often be due to the poor function of the tubes that join the middle ear to the throat – this causes a mild vacuum in the middle ear, stimulating the ear to secrete fluid. This condition may lead to hearing problems.

TREATMENT

Glue ear may sometimes respond to a course of antibiotics but usually it requires the insertion of a grommet, which is a small plastic tube placed through the eardrum by an ear, nose and throat (ENT) surgeon. Grommets allow the pressure between the middle ear and the outer air to equalise, and reduce the secretion of fluid. The grommets usually fall out within three to nine months.

Outer ear infections

Children may also experience infections of the skin of the ear canal on the outside of the eardrum, which is known as otitis externa (meaning 'inflamed outer ear'). This commonly occurs in children who spend a lot of time in water or those with dry skin or eczema of the ear canal.

TREATMENT

Drops containing antibiotics and drugs that act against fungal infections are often used to treat these infections but it is advisable to have an early consultation with an ENT specialist, who may need to clean out the ears working through a microscope.

Drying the ears with cotton buds should be avoided as these may irritate the affected ear even more, and the wool at the end of the bud can come off. Instead, dry ears by shaking the head with the affected ear down. When children have very painful ear infections, sometimes anaesthetic drops can help to reduce the pain – seek advice from your local doctor or pharmacist.

HEARING PROBLEMS

Some babies are born deaf in one or both ears. As they grow older children can also develop hearing problems, most of which are caused by ear infections and glue ear. There are many reasons for deafness in babies, including:

- premature birth (especially if born before 32 weeks)
- the mother contracted an infection, such as rubella (German measles) or CMV (cytomegalovirus), during pregnancy

- genetic disorders (such as Down's syndrome)
- unknown causes – sometimes a cause just cannot be found.

The hearing of all babies should be checked in the first few months of life. If there is any concern about their hearing they will be referred to an audiologist (a hearing specialist), who will carry out more complex hearing testing, and they may also be referred to an ENT specialist to identify a cause for their deafness.

As children get older, hearing problems can be caused by:

- middle ear infection (otitis media)
- glue ear
- meningitis (which can affect many different areas of the brain, and commonly includes the part that controls hearing)
- head injury
- other infections, such as measles, chicken pox and encephalitis, which can, in rare cases, cause hearing problems.

Identifying hearing problems

Children with hearing problems are often slow in developing speech and language skills, including reading and writing. Other signs that children may have a problem with their hearing are if they:

- have difficulty hearing you if they are in another room or when you are driving
- need to turn the television up very loud
- find it difficult to tell which direction a noise is coming from
- show poor performance at school
- have poor vocabulary.

If you have any concerns about your child's hearing, see your local GP and ask for a referral to a paediatrician or ENT specialist.

15

SORE THROATS AND SWOLLEN GLANDS

Sore throats are one of the most common symptoms of childhood disease. Most sore throats will cause swelling of the glands in the neck, but there are some specific conditions that can cause swollen glands that are also important to know about. Diseases commonly associated with sore throats and/or swollen glands are tonsillitis, glandular fever and mumps.

CAUSES OF SORE THROAT

A sore throat (also known as pharyngitis) is often the first thing a child complains of when they are developing a common cold (see Chapter 5: Infections).

Of course, infants will not be able to tell you that they have a sore throat and the only indications you may have that something is wrong is when they display a reluctance to eat or drink, have a fever or a cough, or when the back of their throat may look red (if you can see it).

There are many causes of sore throats in children:

- the common cold
- allergic rhinitis – children with allergies develop runny noses and itchy or sore throats
- indigestion – acid reflux from the stomach can cause a burning pain to the back of the throat
- foreign bodies – fish or chicken bones or other sharp objects stuck in the back of the throat (see Chapter 20: Poisoning and foreign bodies)
- scarlet fever, also known as scarletina – an infection of streptococcus bacteria, which causes fever, swollen red tongue and a rash and is treated with a course of penicillin.

TREATMENT

The vast majority of sore throats are caused by a viral infection that usually resolves itself without treatment, but more serious causes of sore throats include tonsillitis and glandular fever.

Any treatment for sore throats should be aimed at relieving the symptoms with painkillers such as paracetamol or ibuprofen.

You may find that your child will not want to eat; however, you should encourage them to drink plenty of fluids – it may be easier to give small amounts of fluid regularly.

SWOLLEN GLANDS

It is common to get swollen glands in the neck when you have a throat infection. The lymph glands in the neck are part of a network of over a hundred lymph glands or nodes in the body, which are an important part of the immune system (see also page 30). Lymph glands contain large numbers of white blood cells that help in fighting infections and, when you have an infection, the local lymph glands swell with lots of white blood cells working to clear the infection.

It is normal to have swollen glands with an infection as the body fights off the organisms. However, some infections – especially tonsillitis and glandular fever – tend to cause more pronounced lymph gland swelling. The commonest causes of swollen glands in the neck are:

- the common cold
- viral throat infection (including glandular fever)
- bacterial throat infection (including tonsillitis).

Many other infections or inflammations of the head and neck can lead to swollen neck glands. Some of the more common examples are dental infections (for example, tooth abscess), skin infections such as acne or dermatitis, and ear infections (see Chapter 14: Earaches and hearing problems).

TREATMENT

If you are concerned that your child has swollen neck glands and you are not sure what is causing this, you should get an appointment with your GP. The treatment will depend on what your doctor thinks is causing the swollen glands.

TONSILLITIS

Tonsillitis is a form of sore throat that occurs when organisms infect the tonsils. This causes the tonsils to become intensely inflamed, swollen and painful. The tonsils – almond-sized glands at the back of the throat – are part of the immune system like other lymph glands in the body. Adenoids are similar and are located at the back of the nose. Infections of the tonsils or the adenoids can cause some of the other neck glands to become swollen.

Tonsillitis may be caused by viral or bacterial infections. In tonsillitis fever may occur, and the child may complain of feeling hot, cold, shivery and sweaty with muscular aches and pains. It is not usually possible to tell the difference between bacterial and viral tonsillitis from the symptoms alone.

TREATMENT

Antibiotics should only be used when there is evidence of a bacterial infection (doctors may diagnose bacterial infection by using rapid

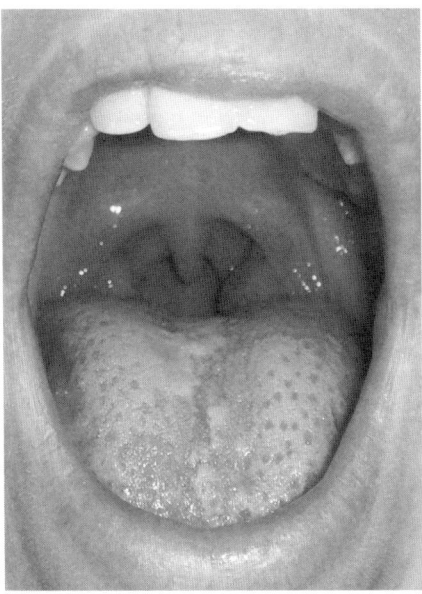

The tonsils are almond-sized glands at the back of the throat.

tests or through clinical judgement based on the length of the disease process). Occasionally the tonsils become so swollen that children may have difficulty swallowing, in which case they may need to be admitted to hospital to have IV antibiotics and fluid drips for a few days until the tonsils are reduced in size and they are feeling better.

Children who get recurrent episodes of tonsillitis, or who have difficulty in breathing or sleeping due to the size of their tonsils, may need to have an operation to remove them (called a tonsillectomy). A common trigger point for performing tonsillectomy is six or more episodes of acute tonsillitis in a single year.

GLANDULAR FEVER

Glandular fever is an acute viral throat infection that also leads to fever, tiredness and enlarged lymph glands in the neck. It is caused by an organism called Epstein-Barr virus, also known as infectious mononucleosis, and is spread mainly by saliva (sharing drinks and so on). Commonly known as the 'kissing disease', as it is usually seen in teenagers and young adults, it can be diagnosed by a blood test.

TREATMENT

Because glandular fever is caused by a virus, antibiotics are not used to treat it. There is no specific treatment – the infection will eventually resolve itself. Sometimes this can take weeks to months and may lead to a form of chronic fatigue syndrome. It is important for your GP to be involved in the follow up, and if the infection is taking a long time to resolve the child may be referred to a paediatrician.

MUMPS

Mumps is a viral infection caused by the mumps virus. It mainly causes swelling of the parotid salivary gland just below the ear, as well as fever, headache and a rash. It is a self-limiting infection and so will resolve itself on its own, but importantly it can affect the testicles in young boys, which subsequently leads to infertility. It can also, but rarely, lead to infections of the brain (meningitis and encephalitis, see page 129).

TREATMENT

A vaccine for mumps is part of the normal MMR (measles, mumps and rubella) vaccination program, so it is becoming a very unusual condition. If you think your child has mumps you should see your GP to confirm the diagnosis.

Mumps is very contagious so you should keep your affected child away from nursery or school. It is not necessary to keep your own children apart because the affected child is infectious before the diagnosis is made. Similarly, there is no need to keep your other children away from school unless they develop symptoms.

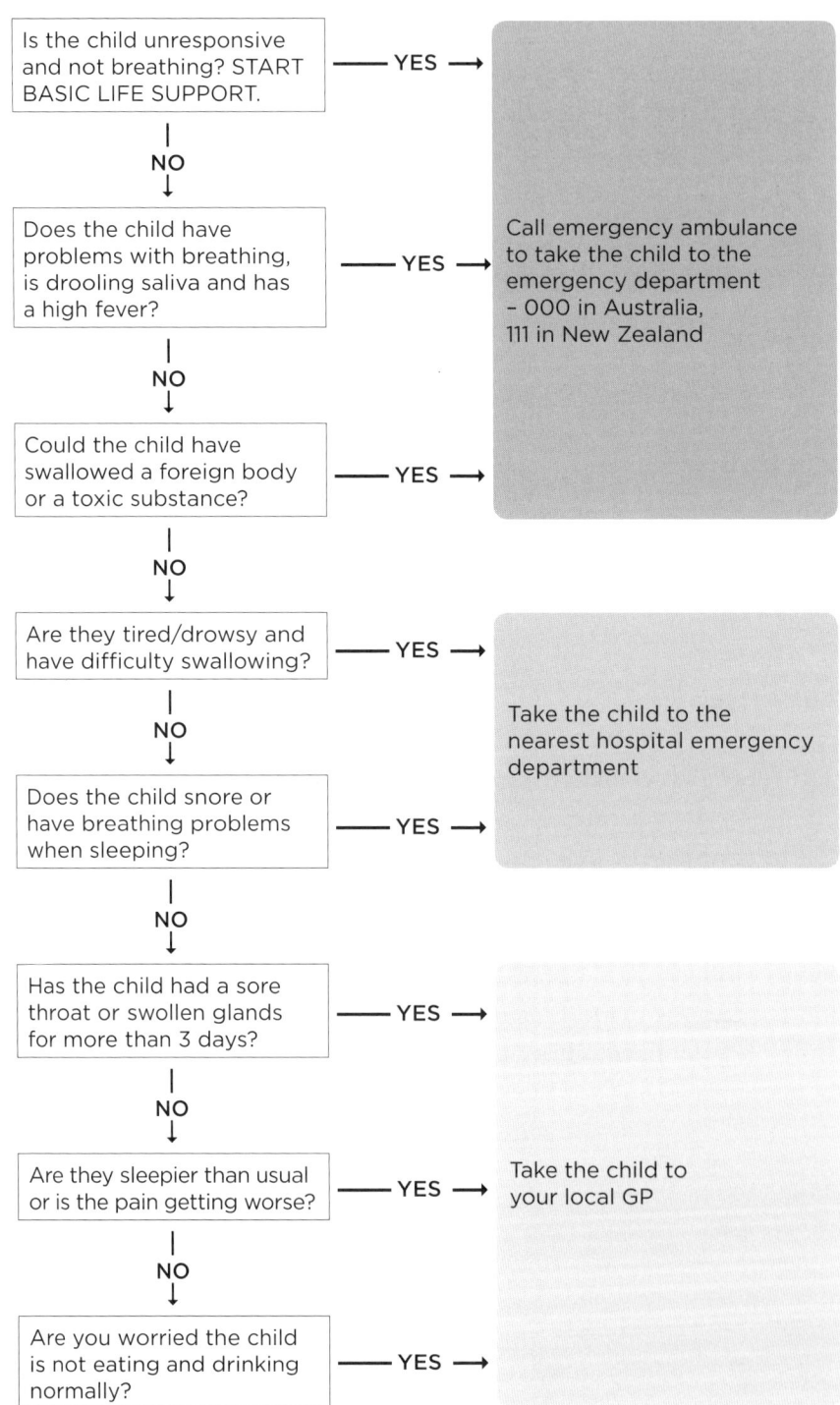

Is the child unresponsive and not breathing? START BASIC LIFE SUPPORT. —— YES →

NO ↓

Does the child have problems with breathing, is drooling saliva and has a high fever? —— YES →

Call emergency ambulance to take the child to the emergency department – 000 in Australia, 111 in New Zealand

NO ↓

Could the child have swallowed a foreign body or a toxic substance? —— YES →

NO ↓

Are they tired/drowsy and have difficulty swallowing? —— YES →

Take the child to the nearest hospital emergency department

NO ↓

Does the child snore or have breathing problems when sleeping? —— YES →

NO ↓

Has the child had a sore throat or swollen glands for more than 3 days? —— YES →

NO ↓

Are they sleepier than usual or is the pain getting worse? —— YES →

Take the child to your local GP

NO ↓

Are you worried the child is not eating and drinking normally? —— YES →

16

MENTAL HEALTH PROBLEMS

The common childhood mental health problems occurring in infancy and early childhood are different from those of the teenage years. Here we explore the signs and symptoms you need to look out for rather than give a detailed account of these mental health conditions or their treatment.

Mental health problems differ from a lot of the physical medical conditions discussed in this book, as most have no 'quick fix'. They tend to require long-term treatment from specialised professionals, including GPs, paediatricians, psychiatrists, psychologists, counsellors and community support groups.

CONDITIONS OF INFANTS AND YOUNG CHILDREN

The mental health problems encountered in infants and young children are usually due to their inability to pay attention, to be 'hyperactive' or very badly behaved. The commonest conditions seen are Attention Deficit Hyperactivity Disorder and autism.

Attention Deficit Hyperactivity Disorder (ADHD)

ADHD is a behavioural rather than a medical condition. It is characterised by a lack of concentration and impulsiveness and is thought to affect 3 to 5 per cent of children in Australia and New Zealand. Some professionals think it is simply one end of the spectrum of normal childhood behaviour. Boys are much more commonly affected than girls. ADHD is a chronic condition which often carries on into adulthood.

The most common signs and symptoms of ADHD are:

- inattention, such as difficulty concentrating, easily distractible, difficulty completing tasks before moving on to something else, difficulty listening
- impulsivity – for example, talking over others, being disorganised, acting before thinking, being accident prone
- hyperactivity, such as fidgeting, being restless, unable to sit still.

Many of these symptoms are shown by all children so the diagnosis can only be made by experienced health professionals. It is important for you as parents to carefully observe your child's behaviour and seek the opinion of carers and teachers. If you think your child may have this disorder seek help from your GP.

Autism

Autism is one of a group of conditions known as Autism Spectrum Disorders (ASD). Other similar conditions in this group are Asperger's syndrome and Pervasive Passive Disorder. Autism usually presents before the age of three years and is a life-long condition. It is characterised by problems with social interaction, restricted and repetitive behaviour and poor communication skills. Autistic children also demonstrate limited imagination and limited ability to play.

It is thought that no two children with this condition exhibit the same combination of problems – this is why it is referred to as a 'spectrum' of disorders. The causes of autism and other ASD are unknown, although it is thought that there may be some genetic, environmental or nutritional factors that play a role.

Sufferers of Asperger's syndrome are considered to be in the more highly functioning part of the spectrum; these children can be very bright but tend to become obsessively interested in only one topic, often to the exclusion of all other activities.

It is difficult to diagnose these disorders. If you are concerned about your child you should seek advice from your GP, who should refer you to a child psychiatrist or specialist paediatrician.

CONDITIONS OF TEENAGE CHILDREN

In the teenage years, different mental health problems tend to arise, such as eating disorders, problems with alcohol and recreational drugs.

Eating disorders

Eating disorders, such as anorexia nervosa and bulimia nervosa, are conditions where a person is obsessed with food and their weight and has a compulsion to either eat or to avoid food. But often the main issue is neither food nor weight but more complex emotional, psychological or social influences. People of all ages can be affected, although the symptoms commonly start in childhood around the age of puberty. The conditions take various forms and have a big impact on the whole of a child's (and their family's) life – physically, emotionally and mentally. Girls are more commonly affected. It is estimated up to two in every hundred teenage girls suffer with an eating disorder.

The management of these disorders is complex and takes a lot of time. All suspected cases of eating disorders should to referred by your GP to a professional who deals in this specialist area: a doctor, nurse or psychologist. There are also many eating disorder support groups and free information on the internet.

ANOREXIA NERVOSA AND BULIMIA NERVOSA

Children with anorexia nervosa have a distorted body image, and try to lose weight to avoid looking or feeling overweight. Bulimia nervosa is similar, but it has a pattern of over-eating followed by purging. To purge, the child causes their body to expel stomach, intestinal or fluid contents through forced vomiting, use of laxatives to increase intestinal excretion (in the stool) or by taking diuretics, which cause increased fluid excretion in the urine. Both anorexia and bulimia can cause very serious medical problems and can even be fatal.

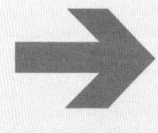

DANGER SIGNS
If you suspect your child of having an eating disorder you should ask your GP or another healthcare professional for referral to expert specialist help.

RECREATIONAL DRUG USE

The drugs commonly used by teenagers and young adults are alcohol, tobacco, cannabis, cocaine, ecstasy, methamphetamine and heroin. If you suspect your teenager is taking drugs talk about it with your GP, who may refer you to the school counsellor or other professional.

Alcohol

This is the most common and probably the most ignored of all drugs of abuse. A depressant that causes relaxation and loss of inhibitions, it is associated with increased sexual activity, violent assault and reckless driving and is one of the leading causes of death in teenagers.

Tobacco

Cigarettes contain the harmful chemicals nicotine, tar and carbon monoxide gas. Nicotine is highly addictive, tar is linked with lung cancer and chronic lung diseases, and carbon monoxide gas is associated with heart disease.

Cannabis

Cannabis – also known as marijuana, hashish, ganja, grass, weed – is a psychoactive drug and is the most commonly used of all the illegal drugs, especially by teenagers. The dried leaves of the cannabis plant are smoked with tobacco. Its use is associated with depression, and in combination with alcohol it has been linked with underage sex. Long-term use is thought to have a negative effect on memory.

Cocaine

Cocaine, a white powder made from the coca plant, is usually snorted (sniffed) but can be smoked or injected. It is a powerful stimulant and highly addictive. Cocaine can affect the heart (causing heart attacks and cardiac arrest), the lungs if smoked ('crack lung'), the brain (the most common cause of strokes in young people) and long term can lead to mental health issues (anxiety, paranoia and aggressive behaviour).

Ecstasy

Methylenedioxymethamphetamine (MDMA or ecstasy) is a stimulant that causes psychedelic hallucinations. Its use is most often associated with all-night dancing (rave parties) in the teenage and young adult population. It can cause hyperpyrexia (abnormally high temperature) and dehydration, due to excess dancing in hot environments and not drinking enough water. It can also lead to drinking too much water, diluting the salts in the blood and body. Both of these conditions can, in extreme circumstances, lead to fitting (convulsions), coma and death. With chronic use there is a known risk of memory loss and muddled thought processing.

Methamphetamine

Also known as 'crystal meth' or 'ice', this highly addictive drug stimulates the brain, causing a heightened sense of awareness, enhancing mood and a general sense of euphoria. If used long term it can affect the heart and brain and lead to severe anorexia and death. Habitual users of methamphetamine will become withdrawn from their friends and family, will avoid previously normal activities (sports, schoolwork), tend to lose weight and develop sores on their skin and in and around their mouths.

Heroin

Heroin (or diamorphine) is related to morphine, a potent painkiller and depressant. Heroin can be injected, smoked or snorted, and has been linked with more illegal drug-related deaths over the years than any other drug. It is highly addictive and can result in severe withdrawal symptoms if not taken regularly.

Signs of potential alcohol or drug use

This can be very difficult because many of the behaviours described are associated with normal healthy teenagers when they are going through the difficult transition from a child to a young adult. Extremes of these behaviours, however, together with evidence of drug taking (pieces of equipment, stories from friends or teachers), may be helpful things to look out for. The signs listed below may suggest that your child is abusing recreational drugs.

When to get help

It is often difficult to gauge whether the child you spend time with every day is displaying behaviour that is normal or abnormal. If you have any concerns you should seek help. The first point of contact is your GP, who can arrange referral to other healthcare professionals. Your child needs to be actively involved in any counselling offered – frank and open discussions (if possible) are very important.

SIGNS OF ALCOHOL OR DRUG USE
At school
- worsening grades, poorer school reports
- loss of interest in sporting activities
- concerned teachers
- truancy.

At home
- changes in friends
- spending more time alone
- more use of perfumes or deodorants (to cover up smells)
- mood swings or changes
- lying about activities/whereabouts
- aggressive behaviour
- unhappiness
- weight gain or weight loss
- money or prescription drugs missing from the household.

PART III

YOUR INJURED CHILD

You need to know what to do when your child has been injured, whether it is a minor trauma or a more serious injury. (Trauma, the medical term for injuries, may be caused by accidents or by intentional violence.) But first it is important to look at how to prevent injuries.

At different ages children are prone to different illnesses (see Chapter 4: How to recognise a seriously ill child). The same is true with injuries. From the age of one, the most common cause of death in children is due to trauma. Most injuries occur because commonsense precautions have not been taken – for example:

- a child falling down stairs that have not been fitted with a gate
- a cup of hot tea left within reach of a toddler
- reckless driving while under the influence of alcohol, causing a motor vehicle accident.

The majority of injuries can be prevented with proper preparation, planning and by thinking ahead.

Most of the time when your child is injured it will be minor. Deaths from accidents occur within three distinct timeframes – immediately, within hours, or days after the accident. Immediate deaths are usually not preventable due to overwhelming injury, and late deaths are usually caused by infections and organ failure in the severely injured while in hospital. The deaths that occur between these two margins are often preventable by prompt and correct action.

Emergency first aid and life-saving intervention during this time – the first couple of hours after serious trauma – can make a huge difference to survival rates and recovery from injury. These interventions may be performed by anyone who knows how – not just by healthcare professionals. Simple but very effective interventions can make a huge difference in the short time period after an injury and are divided into three important actions:

A – opening an unconscious child's **a**irway

B – supporting the **b**reathing of a child

C – putting pressure on any obvious bleeding wounds in an injured child (**C**irculation).

Knowing what to do after your child has suffered a major injury could possibly save their life. What you do really does matter.

17

Injury PREVENTION

Injury is defined as physical harm or damage to the body. It may be caused intentionally or unintentionally. An injury may be minor and require little or no care, or it may be more serious, requiring treatment or hospitalisation, and could result in permanent scarring, disability or death.

Let's look at some statistics.

- Every year in Australia almost two million children under 16 seek medical attention due to injuries.
- Over 50 000 Australian children under 15 years are admitted to hospital due to an injury; this equates to about 160 children each day throughout the country.
- The birth-to-four-years age group are most at risk.
- Falls account for the majority of non-fatal accident.
- In New Zealand poisoning is the second highest cause of hospitalisation in under five year olds.

- Unintentional or accidental injuries account for about 90 per cent of all injury-related deaths in children.
- On average one child dies each day in Australia because of an injury, which is as many childhood deaths as all other causes put together in children older than one year.
- The most common cause of trauma-related deaths in children over five years of age is a motor vehicle accident.
- In Australia and New Zealand the most common cause of death in the under-fives is drowning.

Note that most of these deaths are preventable.

WHY DO CHILDREN HAVE ACCIDENTS?

Children are often absorbed in their own immediate interests so can be oblivious to their surroundings. Because of their lack of experience, they can have a limited perception of the environment and are usually not aware of the potential consequences of the many new situations they encounter daily. Other factors may lead to children being more likely to have accidents than adults.

Small stature This may prevent a child from seeing above and over an obstacle, and their lack of height may make it hard to see them. Small children may not be seen by a car driver, especially when reversing.

Inquisitiveness Curiosity and a spirit of adventure is how children learn about things, but the downside is that it may lead them into danger – simply because they are not aware of the danger.

Bravado and horseplay Boys are particularly prone to showing off and over-reaching their abilities, especially among friends. Many accidents are caused by horseplay involving pushing, shoving and wrestling. Similarly, falls occur when children compete to push the boundaries of their abilities.

Stress Tensions at home and emotional upsets caused by temper, jealousy and over-excitement may cause a child to run blindly into danger. Such action may even be deliberate on the child's part to seek sympathy through attention.

Inexperience A child's interpretation of a situation may be inaccurate, particularly if they have not encountered it previously. Although it is often tempting for adults to believe that children may make the same decisions as they would, carers looking after small children should be aware not to expect too much of them.

Inadequate supervision Children need constant supervision for all the above reasons. Inquisitiveness, a flawed ability to accurately assess risk and the potential for competition among their peers can lead to danger. As part of your supervision you need to ensure medicines, pills and toxic substances are locked away, and heaters, fireplaces, stairs, ovens and other potential danger zones should be guarded.

Safety and child development Children are developmentally unable to appreciate danger. As an example, a child's road safety sense only comes into play after the age of about eight.

WHO HAS ACCIDENTS AND WHEN?

Generally, there is an acknowledged rate of development for children, but individually they do have their own milestones. There are particular ages when accidents are more likely to happen, and social circumstances and gender play a role in this.

- Those aged between birth and four years have the most accidents in the home.
- Boys are more likely to have accidents than girls.
- Childhood injuries are closely linked with social deprivation: children from poorer backgrounds are five times more likely to die as a result of an accident than children from better-off families – and that gap is widening.
- Stress, death in the family, chronic illness, homelessness or moving home increase the likelihood of a child having an accident.

It is also possible to generalise about when and why accidents are more likely to occur.

- Most happen between late afternoon and early evening, in the summer, during school holidays and at weekends.
- Some happen at times of stress, when the usual routine is changed or when people are in a hurry.
- Distractions and inadequate supervision are often the cause of accidents.
- Poor housing and overcrowded conditions are related to increased numbers of accidents.
- Some accidents are caused by a lack of familiarity with surroundings – for example, when visiting relatives or friends or staying in holiday accommodation.

The table opposite, from the British Royal Society for the Prevention of Accidents, breaks down the age groups and their developmental abilities at that age in order to give you some idea of what to do to prevent accidents from happening.

PREVENTING INJURIES

To prevent injuries you need to reduce the chance of them occurring in the first place – for example, by putting up barriers, such as fences around swimming pools or gates at the top of staircases, and avoiding your own risky behaviour such as drink driving.

Prevention of injury is the most useful thing that you, as parents and carers, can do to keep your children safe. Thinking about the potential for injury of whatever sort – at home, at school, on the roads, at the beach – means that actions can be taken to prevent children putting themselves in danger in the first place. This minimises the risk of injury and death and decreases the need for treatment, rehabilitation and any long-term consequences for children and their families.

Safety checklists

A very useful approach to injury prevention is to use safety checklists. Many agencies – including the Children's Hospital Westmead, Sydney

Accidents by ability and prevention method

AGE	ABILITIES	PREVENTATIVE ACTIONS
Up to 6 months	Wriggle and kick, grasp, suck, roll over	Do not leave on a raised surface
6 to 12 months	Stand, sit, crawl, put things in mouth	Keep small objects out of reach
1 to 2 years	Move about, reach high things, find hidden objects, walk, and climb	Never leave alone; place hot drinks out of reach; use a fireguard
2 to 3 years	Be adventurous, climb higher, pull and twist things, watch and copy	Be a good role model and be watchful; place medicines, matches and lighters out of reach
3 to 4 years	Use grown-up things, be helpful, understand instructions, be adventurous, explore, walk downstairs alone	Continue to be a good role model; keep being watchful but start safety training
4 to 5 years	Play exciting games, can be independent, ride a bike, enjoys stories	Continue to be a good role model; continue safety training

Children's Hospital, the Royal Children's Hospital in Melbourne, Kidsafe, the Child Accident Prevention Foundation of Australia and the Child Safety Foundation New Zealand – provide these as downloads from their websites. An example is the Child Health Company's Home Safety Checklist (see page 184). These checklists can be copied and placed in prominent places in the home.

Safety checklists identify potential causes of injury and give pointers to actions that will help to prevent such injury. Burns, choking, drowning, entrapment, falls, poisoning and strangulation can all be caused by predictable events/items. For example, burns can happen because of hot oven doors, hot plates, irons, heaters, hot water taps, hot drinks, chemicals, steam from kettles, open fires, barbeques, candles, matches and the sun. By answering the questions

HOME SAFETY CHECKLIST

The kitchen

- Can you restrict children's access to the kitchen?
- Do you keep electric cords (e.g. kettle/iron) out of reach?
- Do you keep children away from the stove when cooking?
- Do you turn pan handles away from the front of the stove?
- Do you keep hot food and drinks away from the edges of surfaces and tables?
- Do you have a lock on the oven door?
- Do you lock cupboards containing household cleaners?
- Are knives and other sharp objects kept out of reach?
- Is there a fire extinguisher or blanket in or near the kitchen?

General household safety

- Do you stop children playing with electric cords, sockets?
- Do you have safety plugs in your electric sockets?
- Do you keep matches, candles and lighters out of reach?
- Do you put down hot food or drinks when you carry a child?
- Do you cool food and drinks before serving them?
- Do you have fireguards around all fires and heaters?
- Do you have smoke detectors installed in your home?
- Do you regularly check the batteries in smoke detectors and test the alarm function?
- Do you have stair gates?
- Is there secure protective fencing around swimming pools and ponds?
- Do you check pool fences and gates at least once a year?

In the bathroom

- Do you fill the bath with cold water before hot water?
- Do you test the water before putting your child in the bath?
- Do you **always** supervise your child in the bathroom?
- Do you remove all electric appliances from the bathroom?
- Are medicines kept out of the reach?

on the checklists you can identify the interventions you need to put in place. You may even recognise some that are not on the list but are applicable to your home or any place a child may be. For example, 'Do you keep electric cords out of reach?' prompts you to look around and check for situations where your child could be in danger of pulling something down on top of himself.

Some interventions alter the likelihood of injury in situations where accidents may occur. Examples of these are the use of special child seats in cars, cooker and plug guards and cycle helmets. They also include having basic life support and first aid skills (see Chapter 24: Basic life support) to care for injured children if an accident happens.

A useful approach to assessing potential dangers in the home is to:

- spot the hazard
- assess the risk
- fix the problem
- assess the results.

Fitting childproof locks and safety catches on kitchen cupboards makes your home a much safer place for your children.

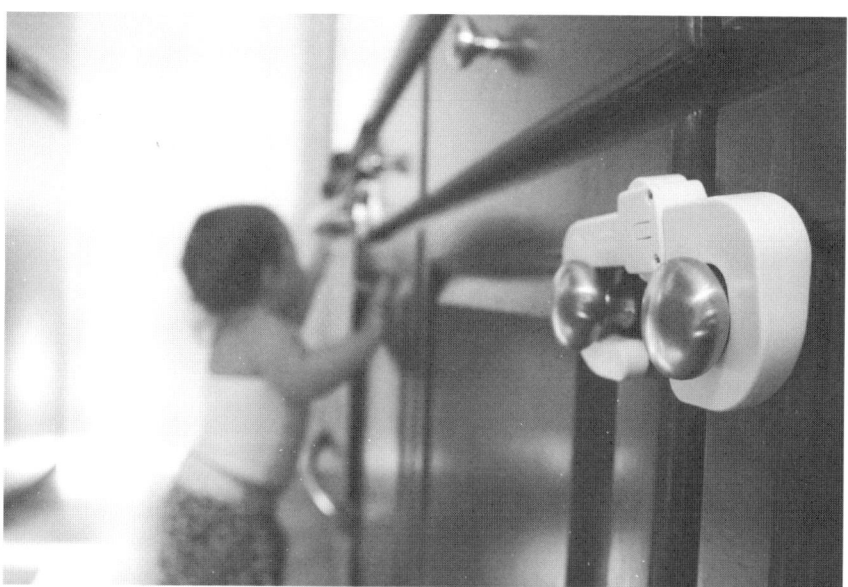

Motor vehicle accidents

Half of all childhood deaths occur as a result of motor vehicle accidents. The use of correctly fitted seat restraints and lap-shoulder harnesses (seat belts) can reduce the incidence of serious injury by 50 per cent.

It is essential that correct age-appropriate car seats and booster seats are fitted for your child – 'capsules' for young babies, car seats for older babies and toddlers, booster seats for older children (see the table below). In the event of a crash, they reduce the risk of children coming out of their seats and either hitting the inside of the car or being ejected from the vehicle. It also reduces stress on small children by keeping them secure when the car is accelerating, braking and cornering. Age-specific car seats and restraints are enforced by law in Australia and New Zealand.

Pedestrian injuries are particularly common in children aged five to nine years, and are usually the result of a child running out into the street and being hit by a car. Although there is no substitute for proper supervision of children, public safety works, such as adequate street lighting and the construction of road barriers for busy roads, are effective in injury prevention. If your street has a particular hazard that can be made safer it might be worth lobbying your local council to ensure your child's wellbeing.

Vehicle restraints

AGE/WEIGHT	RESTRAINT TYPE	COMMENTS
Under 9 months (10 kg)	Rear-facing infant carrier	Do not use with airbag
6 months to 4 years (9–18 kg)	Child seat secured by adult seatbelt	Rear-facing seats now available
4 to 11 years (15–36 kg)	Booster cushion using adult lap and diagonal belt	
Older children	Adult lap and diagonal belt	Both belts better than lap belts alone

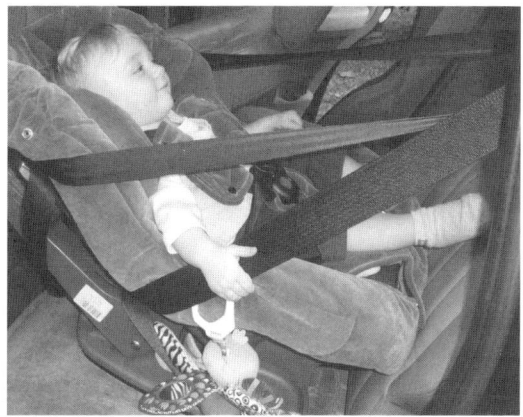

Always use the correct car seats for the child's age and size.

REPLACING CAR SEATS

If they are constantly being put into and removed from cars, child car seats suffer from wear and tear. They should be replaced every five years or according to manufacturers' recommendations. Both child car seats and adult seatbelts in a vehicle that has been involved in a motor vehicle accident should be replaced because they may have suffered damage that is not visible to the naked eye and therefore may not provide adequate protection subsequently.

The use of secondhand child restraints is not advisable, as their prior history (which may include being in a crash) will probably not be known. Secondhand seats are also likely to be older, to have suffered more wear and tear and may not be designed to current safety standards, and it is probable that fitting instructions will be missing.

Bicycle injuries

The majority of serious injuries that result from bicycle accidents are head injuries. The use of cycle helmets reduces the incidence of serious head injury by approximately 80 per cent, but children are still reluctant to use the helmets because they can be uncomfortable

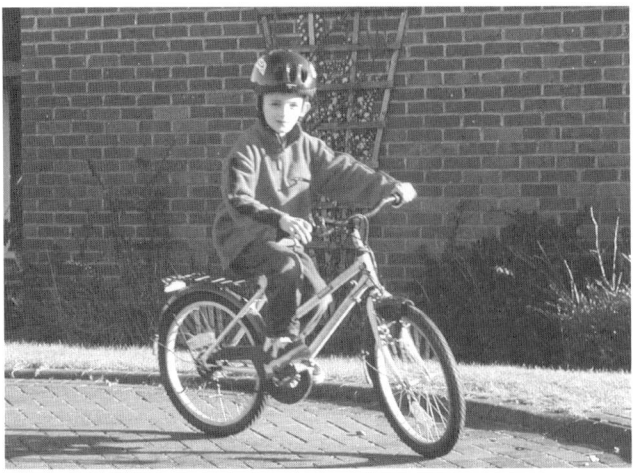

The wearing of cycle helmets is mandatory in Australia and New Zealand. They are designed to protect the head from injury.

and unfashionable. Another contributing factor is the reluctance of parents to wear helmets. For this reason a vigorous education program is ongoing at schools and in the community at large to reinforce the need for, and the effectiveness of, cycle helmets.

A correctly fitted helmet is much more likely to be worn because it will be more comfortable. Therefore, you should ensure that you reassess your child's helmet and replace it as necessary as they grow. However, the most common cause of discomfort, and subsequent reluctance to wear the helmet is catching the child's skin under the chin when clicking the catch shut – so be careful when putting it on.

Drowning

This is a significant cause of death in children, especially in the under-fours. Any water, even a puddle, poses a danger (especially to children with a history of fitting), and they should never be left unattended in bathtubs or near swimming pools, ponds, beaches and rivers.

One of the two most common areas for childhood drowning is the bath – young children should never be left alone in the bath, even for a few seconds. Toddlers and younger siblings are often bathed

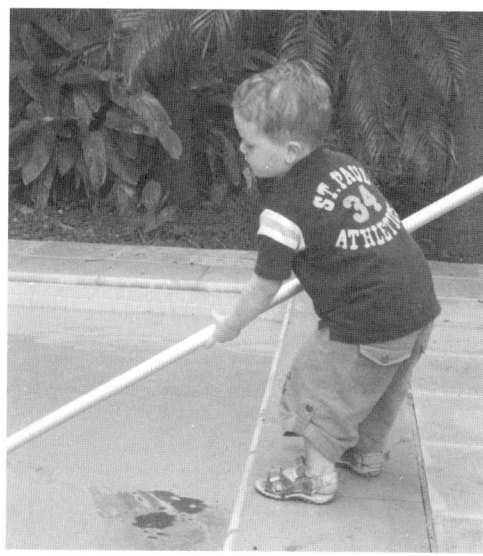

Drowning in residential swimming pools is a significant cause of death for young children. All pools must be fenced and children should never be left unsupervised in or near pools.

together. You need to be aware that young children have no idea of consequences and it only takes four minutes for a child to drown. This may only be as long as answering the phone or boiling a kettle.

Some countries have passed legislation to ensure areas of open water, such as swimming pools, are fenced to prevent unsupervised access to them by children. In Australia and New Zealand all pools must have a child-resistant barrier consisting of fencing or child-safe windows and lockable doors on your house if it opens out onto a pool area. These barriers should be appropriate in height, not encourage climbing, and be checked at least once a year to ensure they are still effective. As children can take great delight in breaking rules, especially those designed to keep them from places that seem exciting, always take your child's abilities into consideration. Be aware that children in your care almost certainly can do far more than you think they can, particularly in terms of climbing.

If a child gets into difficulties in the water, prompt action in the form of basic life support (see Chapter 24) greatly improves the chance of survival. It should be an essential part of your skills, especially if you have a swimming pool or supervise children in any situation near water, including baths.

Burns

House fires account for 80 per cent of deaths caused by burns. Cigarette smoking in the home and the absence of working smoke detectors are both major contributing factors to house fires. Smoking in enclosed spaces, or even out of windows and doors, has been proven to have a harmful effect on children. Preferably, you should stop smoking for your own health, but if you or any of your children's carers do smoke then it should be done outside the house.

Parents and carers of children should ensure they regularly check that smoke detectors are working and replace the batteries, at least on an annual basis. The installation of smoke and carbon monoxide detectors has been shown to reduce the rates of death and injury from house fires. Families should have a planned predetermined escape route from a fire at home.

And you should teach your child about the dangers of playing with fire and matches. Schools often have fire safety programs that are valuable, but don't leave this important aspect of your children's education to someone else. Make sure they know the risks.

Again, safety checklists will provide you with excellent guidelines to assess your home and to put in place preventative measures to ensure the lowest risk of burn injury. Discuss this with your local fire brigade or access its website for a relevant safety checklist for your area. This is particularly important in bushfire-prone areas.

Poisoning

Poisoning in young children often results from eating dishwasher tablets, drinking household cleaners or garden fluids such as pesticides and weedkillers, and swallowing medications or supplements not suitable for children. Many of these are highly toxic and can easily cause a child's death. As with most hazards, the strategies to prevent poisoning largely involve commonsense interventions.

- All toxic fluids, such as weedkillers and household cleaners, should be kept in well-marked containers.
- Toxic fluids should never be put in bottles that once held drinks such as cordials – children may think they are safe to drink.

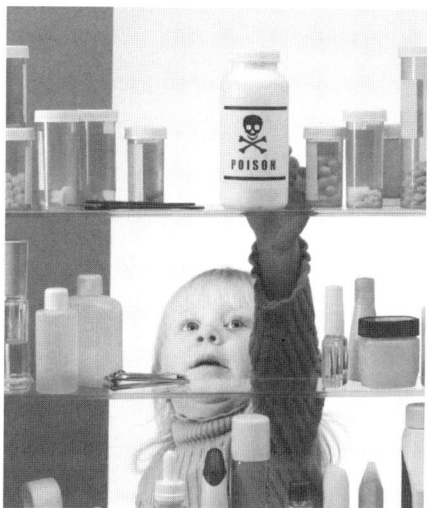

Medicine cabinets should be fitted with childproof locks.

- All potentially harmful materials should be stored high on a shelf or in a cupboard.
- Any outhouses or sheds should be kept locked and secure, preferably with a self-closing and locking mechanism.
- Within the house, particularly in the kitchen and bathroom, household cleaners and powders should be kept in a single, lockable cupboard, preferably in a high place.
- All locks on cupboards and drawers should be childproof, and parents and carers need to be scrupulous in their attention to shutting and locking these areas. Simple drawer and cupboard locks may be purchased in hardware shops reasonably inexpensively; an alternative is to tie cupboard doors with string or some other securing mechanism.

Unsafe buildings

Building and demolition sites exert a fascination on children. These areas are a clear risk to the inquisitive child – unsafe footing, falling masonry and sharp objects can all cause injury. If you are undergoing renovations, these areas should be made secure from trespass and warning signs should be clearly displayed. You should also ensure your child knows not to enter building sites.

18

INJURIES
AND TRAUMA

The ABC (airways, breathing and circulation) assessment technique, used when dealing with a child who is ill (see page 252), is also used for an injured child – but there are some significant differences. Prompt treatment of injuries at the scene of accidents may be life saving and can reduce the complications that may result from trauma. You will also be dealing with more minor injuries such as falls and bumps, as children run into things and hurt themselves all the time on an almost everyday basis, so it is useful to have some knowledge of how to deal with them.

When a child has sustained an injury, prompt assessment and emergency first aid are crucial. Failure to adequately ensure the child has an open airway in the first hour after an injury has been shown to be a major cause of preventable deaths. This first hour is known as the 'golden hour', because it is during this time that life-saving treatments will be most effective. Treating children who have sustained an injury can be more difficult than treating adults with similar problems –

partly because children become very frightened and may not be able to communicate the exact nature of their injuries, and they are less able to understand what has happened to them.

WHAT TO DO FIRST

Start with checking the child's airway, breathing and circulation, and then evaluating the injuries in more detail. However, after an injury has occurred, there are other specific checks that need to be done.

Check airway, keeping cervical spine immobile

The cervical spine is the part of the backbone that makes up the back of the neck. This is a particularly vulnerable part of the anatomy because it is delicate and flexible, and it also has the job of supporting the head. The other end of this flexible piece of spine is firmly attached to the structures of the chest; the ribs, sternum and spine form a rigid cage. This structure – a heavy head at one end with the bottom end of the neck being fixed – creates great potential for damage in this area of the body.

The cervical spine is most commonly injured as a result of a fall from a height or a high-speed motor vehicle accident. It may also be damaged in association with severe injuries to the head or face. Missing a spinal injury can have tragic consequences, so it should be assumed that a child who has sustained trauma has a neck injury until proven otherwise.

The most important thing to do is keep the child still – any movement may worsen their condition and could result in long-term paralysis or even death.

When checking the airway (as described on page 254) a head-tilt/chin-lift procedure should not be performed because this may

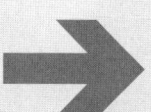

SERIOUS INJURY CAUTION
Any child sustaining serious trauma should be assumed to have a neck and back injury until this has been excluded by doctors in the hospital.

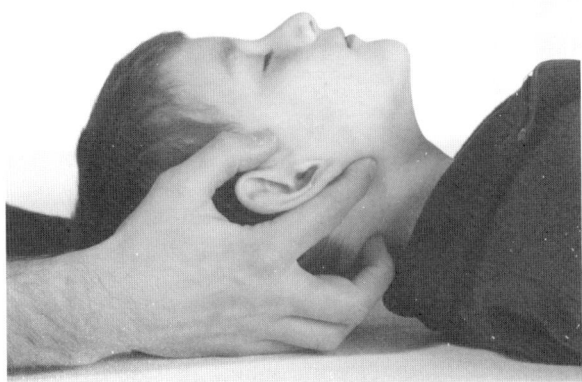

In the jaw thrust manoeuvre, the head and neck are held in a straight line, and the airway is opened by pushing the jaw forwards with the fingers.

worsen a spinal injury. If the airway needs to be opened or cleared it should be done by the jaw thrust manoeuvre, which does not involve moving the neck.

Support the head in line with the body using your hands and forearms by placing a hand on each side of the child's head and holding the head still, in line with the body (see the photograph above). In a patient who is unconscious you may need help from someone else to perform the jaw thrust if the airway is not open; if you are alone and the airway is obstructed, then apply the jaw thrust but try not to move the neck.

In a conscious child who may be in a lot of pain, especially if distressed and moving about, you may have great difficulty in protecting them from any potential spine injury. If you apply force to keep the spine straight, there is often more movement from the child as a result and increased distress for them.

You need to start by offering reassurance and comfort. Bear in mind, if the child is conscious and requires comforting then the airway is usually open. Lie beside the child and maintain the head and neck position with a combination of encouragement and physical support.

With smaller babies and toddlers, the position can often be maintained by holding them between your arms on your front with the head at breast level.

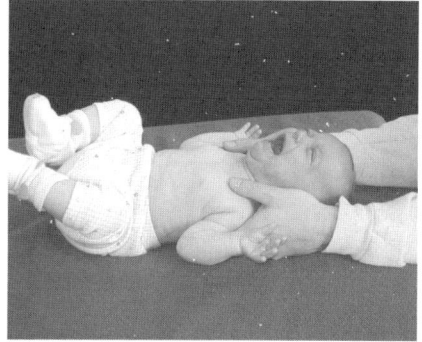
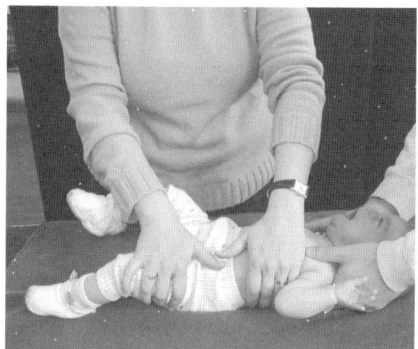
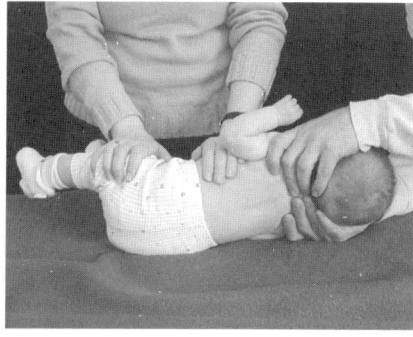

Demonstrating spinal care for the injured baby – the head and body are moved as one by supporting the head on the shoulders.

It may be possible to keep the child completely still if they are very cooperative and/or after analgesia are given when emergency services arrive. In every situation, aim for the best immobilisation you can provide. This is very important, as the best way to prevent worsening of any spinal injury is by making sure there is no or minimal movement of the head and neck.

A screaming child is distressing for anyone to deal with, and if you panic it will not improve the situation. However, if a child is crying and talking, at least this tells you that they have a clear airway and are breathing. Therefore, the first and second parts of the assessment of the injured child are complete before they have even been touched.

Check breathing

Your child's breathing should be assessed as described in 'Basic life support' (see Chapter 24). If the child is not breathing, then mouth-to-mouth resuscitation should be commenced (see page 257).Injuries to the chest may increase the work of breathing or make it very painful for the child to breathe, which is important to note and to describe to the paramedics or other emergency services.

Check circulation and control bleeding

Part of circulation assessment and management includes the control of any bleeding, especially from any external wounds.

Most wounds will stop bleeding if direct pressure is applied through a clean dressing and the affected area elevated if possible. The direct pressure should be for at least five minutes or longer.

In very large bleeds apply pressure and do not remove it until there is a good reason, such as a doctor being ready to inspect the wound or somebody else taking over the pressure position for you.

Do not look at the wound every few minutes to check if the bleeding has stopped. If you keep taking a look at the wound you can allow a lot of precious blood to be lost, and an open wound is vulnerable to infection.

Any obvious haemorrhage should be stopped as soon as practically possible, because ongoing bleeding may cause major problems and even death. Ideally, some sort of clean material should be used as a pad to press on a bleeding area, but if none is available then any item of clean clothing or other material will do.

Check the patient's pulse and skin colour. In the event of trauma the circulation is commonly affected by loss of blood, which makes the pulse rate go up and may make the skin appear pale and sweaty. Blood may be lost via an obvious point of bleeding such as a cut, but it may also be lost internally – into the chest or abdomen if an organ is damaged, or into the soft tissues surrounding a bone if the bone is broken. Internal injuries may not always be obvious.

You will need to maintain a high degree of suspicion that there may be internal injury, especially in children. In adults, the ribcage is quite rigid and a certain force has to be applied to break a rib – therefore a broken bone may provide a clue as to the amount of underlying damage to internal organs such as the lungs. In children, however, the ribcage is quite elastic and can sustain the same force without breaking the bones. This means you cannot assume that the underlying internal organs have not been damaged – even if there appears to be no apparent damage. The internal organs, such as the liver and the spleen, are comparatively larger in a child's body than an adult, so they are more easily injured.

The risk of internal organ damage is particularly high following certain types of injury, such as car accidents or falls from a significant height. The elasticity in children's bones also means – if there is localised pain, bruising and the suspicion of a broken rib – that the likelihood of underlying lung damage is increased substantially, more than would be expected in adults.

Accidents involving a car hitting a child are particularly dangerous, as the car bumper, grille and headlights (which would damage the legs, knees or hips in an adult) will impact on a child's abdomen and chest and on all the essential organs contained in this area.

DO A MORE DETAILED EXAMINATION

Following your initial assessment, a more detailed examination of the child will reveal the precise nature of the injuries sustained.

The following sections deal with trauma to various parts of the body and how to check them, but you should always assume that more than one part of the body might be injured.

SIGNS OF NEED FOR MEDICAL ATTENTION AFTER INJURY
- Penetrating injury
- Loss of consciousness
- Undue drowsiness, not fully responsive afterwards
- Vomiting
- Visual disturbance
- Severe headache, convulsions or weakness
- Painful or stiff neck.

Head injuries

Children often fall and bang their heads. Most of these injuries are minor bumps and bruises that require no further treatment or investigation. It is a particularly common thing to happen with toddlers, when they are just starting to find their feet and seem to bump into things on a regular basis. Serious head injuries are most commonly associated with motor vehicle accidents and falls from a significant height (for example, from a tree or a window). Compared with injuries to other parts of the body, though, head injuries from accidents cause the greatest number of deaths.

There are some important factors you need to consider when assessing a child with a head injury:

- the force of the injury – if a child has been hit by a car, for example, the head injury is likely to be more serious than if they have bumped their head on a cupboard door
- whether the child lost consciousness – if they cried immediately, they are unlikely to have been knocked out
- when they regained full consciousness if knocked out
- the events immediately after the head injury – for example, did they act normally, vomit, have a seizure, or develop any weakness of the limbs
- any evidence of a penetrating injury (a wound)
- the child's recollections before and after the event.

Once the above factors have been established, the potential seriousness of the head injury can be judged. If any of the signs listed in the box on page 197 occurred an urgent medical opinion should be sought, and the child should be transported to hospital immediately via an ambulance. Call 000 in Australia, 111 in New Zealand.

PREVENTING FURTHER INJURY
The damage done to the brain in serious head injury may be both primary and secondary. Primary damage occurs at the time of injury as a result of direct trauma. Secondary damage occurs after the event – for example, from lack of oxygen to the brain due to an obstructed airway or insufficient blood pressure to get the oxygen there.

The treatment of serious head injuries is aimed at avoiding any worsening of the situation. The first step is to call an ambulance and

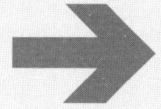

AIRWAYS, SPINE, BREATHING

It is important to remember that in almost all cases, problems with airway, cervical spine alignment and breathing take precedence over the bleeding from a head wound (even though that is a circulation problem).

The possible exception may be in a small child, infant or baby, where there might be sufficient bleeding from a head wound to cause problems in its own right.

evaluate the child's airways, breathing and circulation – as with any seriously injured patient.

You should make sure the airway is open – remembering to control the cervical spine and keep it in a straight line (see page 193) – checking that breathing is adequate, and then checking circulation and controlling any bleeding.

If any problems are identified, they must be dealt with immediately while waiting for the ambulance – but there should be no delay in getting the child with a serious head injury to hospital.

If there is a bleeding head wound, direct firm pressure should be applied to the wound through a clean dressing. This will stop the bleeding in the majority of wounds but may take a prolonged period of pressure to be successful. A bleeding head wound should be reviewed by a doctor, nurse or paramedic, who is able to decide if the wound should be closed with stitches or an alternative method is required.

If the head injury is of a more minor nature, then a decision should be made whether to seek a medical opinion. If none of the factors mentioned in the box on page 197 apply and the child is well, they may be observed closely at home and given simple pain relief such as paracetamol or ibuprofen to relieve any headache. If any of the symptoms listed in the box do develop a medical opinion should be sought urgently.

Injuries to the chest and abdomen

Trauma to the torso can range from a trivial bruise to major internal injuries. A similar approach to that outlined for head injuries must be used to define who needs to be seen in hospital and who can be observed at home.

Significant trauma to the torso is usually a result of a road traffic accident or a fall from a great height. However, due to their more flexible ribcage, the contents of children's abdomen and chest have less protection and they may be injured more easily. Therefore, you need to maintain a high degree of suspicion so that potentially serious injuries are not overlooked.

Bruising on the abdomen is especially concerning. Children have very weak, thin abdominal wall muscles. Any trauma that has sufficient force to cause a bruise on a child's abdomen may have also caused some internal damage. In this case, seek advice from a hospital's emergency department.

The absence of bruising after abdominal injury does not exclude possible serious internal injury. If your child complains of pain in the chest or abdomen or has difficulty breathing, then a medical opinion should be sought urgently.

Children who have suffered serious torso injuries (see below) should be taken to hospital, especially if they are feeling any pain or discomfort.

SERIOUS TYPES OF TORSO INJURIES

Any injuries sustained by the following means need immediate medical attention:

- significant road traffic accidents – as pedestrian, cyclist or passenger in a car
- crush injuries – for example, rolled on by a horse following a fall
- penetrating injuries
- falls from a significant height.

SOME DEFINITIONS

A **fracture** is the medical term for a broken bone. A **break** and a fracture are exactly the same thing and the words can be used interchangeably.

A **bruise** is caused by bleeding under the surface of the skin. Bruises start off pink or red and, as the blood becomes old and is slowly absorbed by the body, they change colour to purple, black, green and yellow. Bruises are usually caused by a blunt force injury to the skin. The medical term for a bruise is a **contusion**.

Cuts are breaks in the surface of the skin due mostly to blunt trauma (such as falling and hitting your head on the ground), called 'lacerations'; or to a sharp injury (made with a scalpel during a surgical procedure), called 'incisions' or 'incised wounds'.

When the surface of the skin is scraped (after a fall onto a road or carpet) the injury is called an **abrasion** (or 'graze'). These injuries occur when only the top layer of skin is breached. Abrasions can ooze with blood or lymph (clear fluid often seen coming from the wound in these types of injuries).

After injuries such as a sprained ankle or a kick to the shin a **swelling** (or **haematoma**) may occur. A haematoma is a bruise or collection of blood deeper under the surface of the skin (for example, in the soft tissues, muscles or ligaments).

Injuries to the limbs

If a child has multiple injuries, the injuries to the head and torso usually take priority. This is because it is very unusual for a limb injury to be life threatening and its medical care can be delayed until other more urgent treatment is carried out. Exceptions to this rule are where there is traumatic amputation of a limb and broken long bones such as the femur (thigh bone).

A broken femur can bleed into the surrounding tissues of the thigh, resulting in a loss of about a fifth of the body's blood volume. If there is more than one broken bone or if the broken ends can be seen outside the skin, the situation is serious because even more blood loss may occur. In any situation where there is no immediate medical help for a child injured in this way, the best thing that can be done is to immobilise the limb, keeping it as still as possible.

Even in cases of multiple injuries, the structured approach of checking the airways, breathing and circulation first should still be followed so a more serious or life-threatening problem is not missed.

Minor injuries

The most common reason to take children to a hospital emergency department is a fall. As infants become mobile and begin to explore their environments, and because they are unsteady on their feet and lack insight into the possible outcome of their actions, they fall. The majority of these injuries are minor and require little, if any, treatment. The most frequently seen minor injuries are broken bones, bruises, cuts and sprains and strains.

BROKEN BONES

Specific types of breaks that affect children, called 'greenstick' fractures, are a result of the flexibility of children's bones. These typically occur when one side of the bone deforms or buckles without breaking completely. Greenstick fractures – named because the break is incomplete and looks similar to a young tree branch when broken – are more common in the forearm and wrist, but can also occur in other bones. On an x-ray bones show up as white, and skin and other soft tissues are grey or black.

The treatment of suspected broken limbs is based on aligning and immobilising the limb and this is something you can do. If there has been a fracture to a bone, gentle pulling (traction) on the limb to realign it back to its normal position will ease the pain and reduce bleeding from the fractured site. Even if you are reluctant or unable to

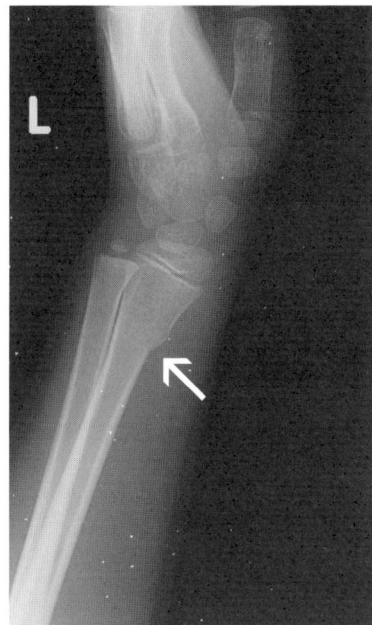

An x-ray showing a 'greenstick' fracture of a child's arm.

attempt to gently pull on a probable fractured limb, immobilising it with any sort of splint will act as very effective pain relief. The affected bone is splinted, either against an adjacent bone (for example, taping two fingers together) or against something rigid, such as a plaster cast or a stick. Immobilising the limb like this reduces movement at the fracture site and the amount of discomfort felt by the child. If a medical splint is available it should be used, but any rigid object can be used as a makeshift device.

If the limb is one of many injuries you should call an ambulance immediately, but if it is an isolated injury and the child is well and coping, then you should go to an emergency department (or to your GP if you are some distance from the hospital) as soon as possible.

Applying ice to the affected area and elevating the injured part may reduce swelling and help restore normal function to a fractured limb. To apply ice, make a cool pack out of a bag of crushed ice (or a packet of frozen food), cover the affected limb with a damp towel and over that apply the cool pack (which should not be in direct contact with the skin). Then wrap the packed limb in a dry towel, elevating

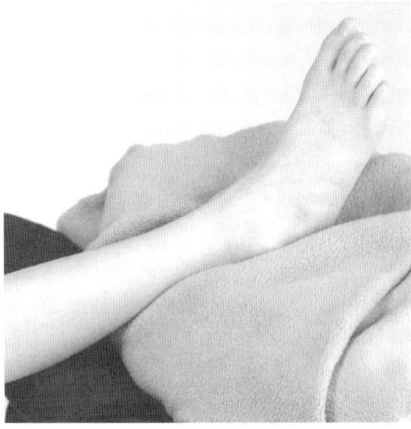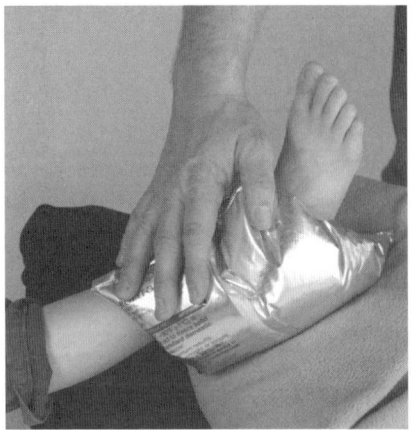

Elevating the limb and applying an ice pack (making sure that the ice is not directly touching the skin) helps prevent swelling.

the limb if possible. Leave the cool pack in place for 10 to 20 minutes and repeat the process three or four times a day.

BRUISING

Bruises are common – in fact, much more common than cuts or abrasions. Toddlers frequently have multiple bruises on their legs due to repeated falls and walking into objects. Most of these bruises are of little significance and will fade with time. Some bruises, though, can overlie more serious injuries. Broken bones (or fractures) will frequently have a bruise associated with them. If your child has bruising, is in pain and is not using the part of the body affected, they may have a fracture – you should take them to your GP or an emergency department for evaluation.

Bruising on the abdomen is a very important sign that your child needs to be assessed by a medical professional (see Injuries to the chest and abdomen, page 200, for more details).

CUTS

The first aid treatment for cuts (lacerations) is to stop the bleeding first. To do this, use a clean bandage and apply pressure to the wound with it, elevating the limb if possible (see Check circulation and control bleeding, page 196, for more detail). If the cut is serious it should be assessed by a doctor or nurse to see if it needs to be stitched or closed with other techniques. These days there are many different techniques for wound closure, such as adhesive strips ('paper stitches') and wound glue ('tissue adhesive'), which are easier than stitching and therefore more acceptable to children and parents alike.

Small superficial cuts in which the edges are touching together with no further bleeding can be managed with cleaning and dressing at home if you have the correct equipment. First, clean the cut. The best way to do this is by gentle cleansing with clean gauze or cotton wool balls soaked in cold tap water. (There is good medical evidence to show that using tap water to clean wounds is as effective as antiseptic solutions or iodine.) After cleaning, the cut should be covered with a watertight dressing (see Appendix I: Your home medicine cabinet).

Abrasions should be cleaned in the same way, with attention paid to removing any pieces of foreign material in the wound, as these may lead to infection. A good non-stick dressing is preferred for abrasions.

You should always ensure your child is up to date with their tetanus immunisation (see page 77). If you are not sure about this talk to your GP, who will hold your child's records and will know when their last tetanus shot was administered. Tetanus (sometimes called 'lock-jaw') is caused by the bacteria *Clostridium tetani*, found in dust and animal faeces. Infection may occur even after minor injury. Although the disease is fairly uncommon now, it can be fatal.

SPRAINS AND STRAINS

Sprains and strains are injuries of the body's soft tissues, such as a tear of a ligament, tendon or muscle. Although these injuries are common they should still be taken seriously, because they are potentially very painful and symptoms may last for several weeks if they are not treated correctly. These injuries tend to produce a swelling or haematoma over the site.

The treatment for sprains and strains is similar to that for broken bones. Applying ice to the affected area and elevating the limb will reduce swelling and improve function. The area should always be checked to ensure that it is returning to normal colour. A compression bandage may also be used to reduce swelling. An initial short period of rest should be followed by gentle exercise – as much as the pain will allow.

Simple painkillers such as paracetamol and ibuprofen will ease the pain from such an injury and allow gentle use of the limb; however, anti-inflammatory drugs such as ibuprofen should not be taken by patients with asthma or stomach ulcers unless advised to do so by a doctor who is aware of the condition.

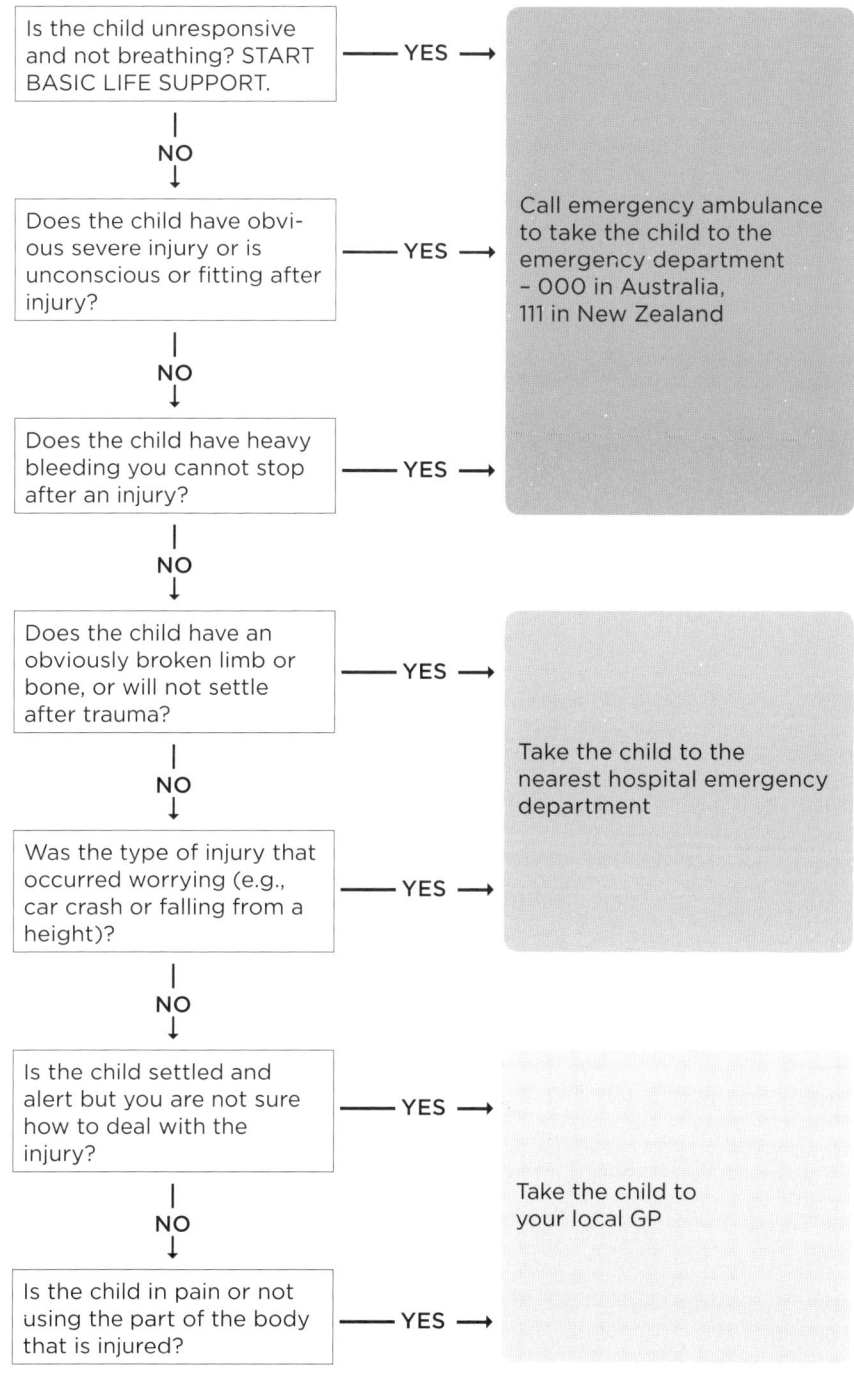

Is the child unresponsive and not breathing? START BASIC LIFE SUPPORT. — YES →

NO ↓

Does the child have obvious severe injury or is unconscious or fitting after injury? — YES →

NO ↓

Does the child have heavy bleeding you cannot stop after an injury? — YES →

Call emergency ambulance to take the child to the emergency department – 000 in Australia, 111 in New Zealand

NO ↓

Does the child have an obviously broken limb or bone, or will not settle after trauma? — YES →

NO ↓

Was the type of injury that occurred worrying (e.g., car crash or falling from a height)? — YES →

Take the child to the nearest hospital emergency department

NO ↓

Is the child settled and alert but you are not sure how to deal with the injury? — YES →

NO ↓

Is the child in pain or not using the part of the body that is injured? — YES →

Take the child to your local GP

19

BURNS
AND SCALDS

Children suffer burns and scalds more frequently than adults do, and children's skin is also more sensitive so it scars more readily than adults. The fact that children are inquisitive, like to explore their local environment and may not know that hot drinks and hot water can burn may lead to their higher risks of sustaining these injuries. Fortunately, though, the incidence of serious and disfiguring burns has decreased over the last 20 years due to better awareness of its causes and likelihood.

A combination of factors has led to the decreasing incidence of fatal and severe burns. These include the introduction of smoke alarms, homes having fewer open fires, the education of parents regarding the dangers of fires and heaters and the use of fireguards, and stringent measures to ensure the fire safety of household furniture and clothing. The majority of deaths due to 'burn' injury, however, are caused by smoke inhalation from house fires, and these are mostly preventable (see Chapter 17: Injury prevention).

TYPES OF BURNS

A burn is any damage to the skin that occurs due to hot liquids and contact with hot solids, flames, fires or chemicals. A scald is a specific type of burn caused by hot liquids or by steam. Most minor burns are scalds caused by hot liquids such as tea or coffee. Those caused by hot bath water and cooking fat are also common. Flame burns occur more often in older children.

The severity of injury depends on various factors:

- temperature
- the length of exposure to that temperature
- the type of burning material involved.

For example, at over 70°C a significant burn can result from just a one-second contact, whereas at 50°C it may take up to a minute before injury occurs. On top of that, the size of the area of the body that is burned or scalded is extremely important. A large burn will have a greater effect on the body's systems – for example, there will be a great loss of fluid from the injury.

Grading burns

The area of a burn is judged as a percentage of the total body surface area. For instance, the surface of a child's palm is approximately 1 per cent of their body surface.

In hospitals, burn areas are assessed by standard body charts that calculate the percentage of skin surface that has been burned. This is very important information because it helps with the subsequent management of the burn by allowing doctors and nurses to work out how much fluid needs to be replaced to bring the body back to normal and prevent further complications.

Burns are also graded into categories, depending on the depth of tissues that are affected:

- Burns that cause some redness, with no other problems, are 'superficial' (mild sunburn is a good example).
- Burns that penetrate deeper into the skin and underlying tissues

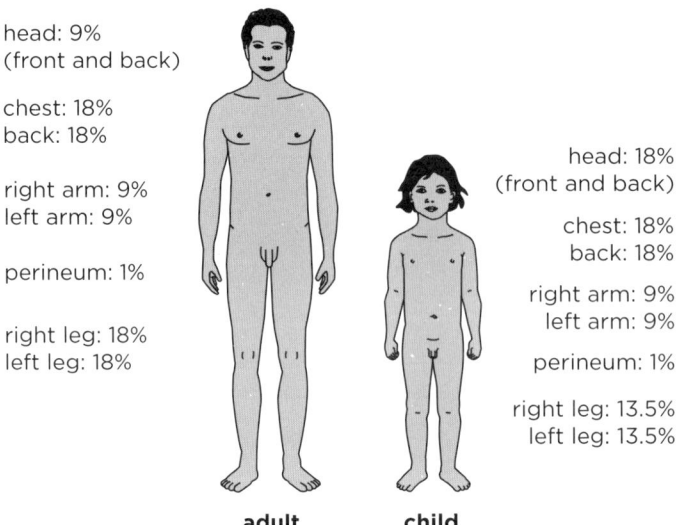

head: 9%
(front and back)

chest: 18%
back: 18%

right arm: 9%
left arm: 9%

perineum: 1%

right leg: 18%
left leg: 18%

head: 18%
(front and back)

chest: 18%
back: 18%

right arm: 9%
left arm: 9%

perineum: 1%

right leg: 13.5%
left leg: 13.5%

adult　**child**

Clinicians use burns charts to calculate the size of the area that has been burned and, thus, the best method of treating the injury. Charts for adults and children are different because the proportions of their bodies are different.

are graded as either 'partial thickness' or 'full thickness', and will have blistering or the burned skin will look white or black in colour.

These categories help with emergency care. It allows the potential severity of burns and scalds to be estimated and the information is then easy to accurately pass between emergency services – from an ambulance officer to an emergency department doctor to another emergency department doctor to the burns unit doctor, and so on.

FIRST AID FOR TREATING BURNS

Follow these steps to treat burns:

- put the burned area under cool running water
- cover the affected area
- provide pain relief.

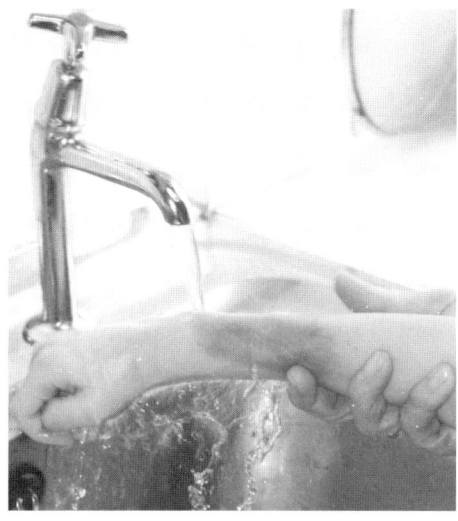

It is important to place the burned area under cold running water as soon as possible.

The injury needs to be placed under cool running water for 20 minutes. This is vital because it initially reduces the temperature of the burned area and also has biochemical effects that may prevent the injury becoming more severe. It is important not to do this for longer than 20 minutes, especially with large burned areas, because excessive heat loss may occur. This is particularly the case with children because of their tendency to lose heat quite quickly (see Chapter 1: How the body works). Too much cooling can cause hypothermia. For the same reason, it is also important not to put wet dressings such as towels soaked in cold water on the injury.

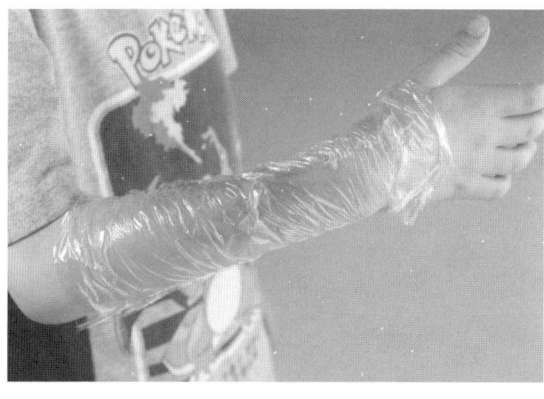

Once the burn has been cooled, cover it with a clean non-stick dressing. Plastic clingfilm is ideal.

During or after the 20 minutes, remove rings or other jewellery and burned clothing that is not sticking to the burn. Then reduce the air flow over the affected area – the pain experienced from these injuries is not just due to the burn but also to the movement of air over the surface of the burned area.

The area should be covered with a clean non-sticking dressing, applied so it is touching but not tight. Kitchen clingfilm is ideal for this purpose; if that is not available, a clean sheet may be used. Blisters should be left intact if possible. Once the wound is covered, pain relief such as paracetamol or ibuprofen should be administered.

ASSESSING CHILDREN WITH BURNS OR SCALDS

Many severely burned children will also have other injuries that need attention. A structured approach to assessing them is needed to ensure no injuries are missed. The initial management should follow the same airway, breathing and circulation assessment used in trauma assessment (see Chapter 18: Injuries and trauma). This will ensure more serious injuries are not missed because you are concentrating on the burn.

Most deaths associated with burns are the result of inhaling smoke, so it is paramount to ensure the injured child has an open airway. Breathing should be assessed next, before moving on to anything else. A child with burns to the face, or inside the mouth or nose, or with any changes in their voice such as hoarseness, needs urgent attention at a hospital as there is an immediate danger of their airway being obstructed because of swelling of the burnt tissues. Call an ambulance.

After checking airways and breathing, the child's circulation should be monitored (by checking for a pulse).

Oxygen is an important treatment for smoke inhalation and will be administered as soon as the ambulance crew arrives. Smoke contains poisonous substances including carbon monoxide, a colourless, odourless gas that removes vital oxygen from the haemoglobin in the blood so the body's cells and tissues cannot be supplied with enough oxygen to function. The best way to get rid of this poisonous gas from the blood is to increase the concentration of inhaled oxygen, which will then displace the carbon monoxide. At a minimum, the child should be removed from any area that still has smoke in the air.

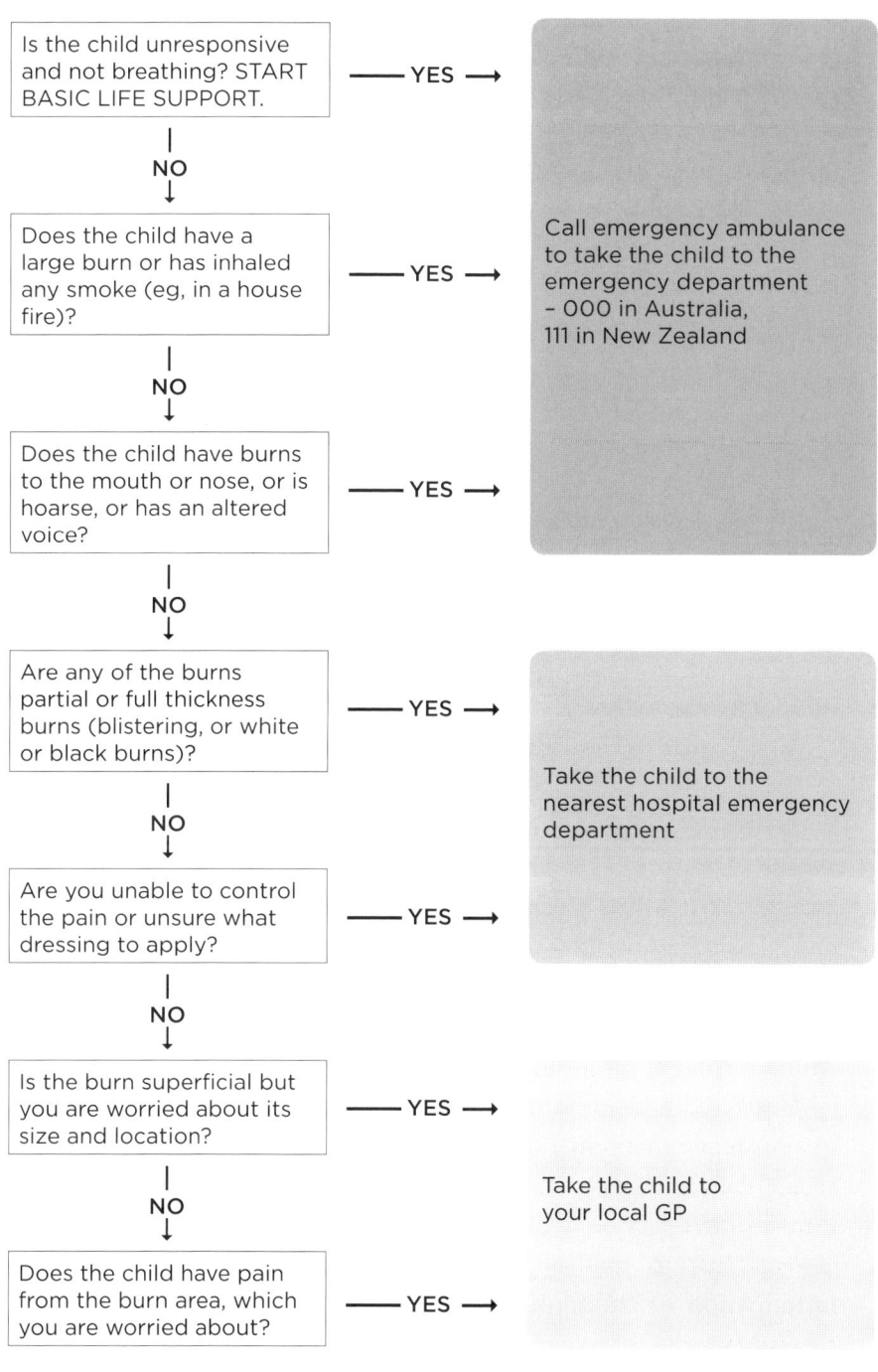

Is the child unresponsive and not breathing? START BASIC LIFE SUPPORT.

— YES →

NO ↓

Does the child have a large burn or has inhaled any smoke (eg, in a house fire)?

— YES →

NO ↓

Does the child have burns to the mouth or nose, or is hoarse, or has an altered voice?

— YES →

Call emergency ambulance to take the child to the emergency department – 000 in Australia, 111 in New Zealand

NO ↓

Are any of the burns partial or full thickness burns (blistering, or white or black burns)?

— YES →

NO ↓

Are you unable to control the pain or unsure what dressing to apply?

— YES →

Take the child to the nearest hospital emergency department

NO ↓

Is the burn superficial but you are worried about its size and location?

— YES →

NO ↓

Take the child to your local GP

Does the child have pain from the burn area, which you are worried about?

— YES →

20

POISONING
AND FOREIGN BODIES

Unfortunately, part of a child's normal development is to pass through a stage of putting everything they can lay their hands on into their mouth. This is fine most of the time, but can cause problems if it involves objects or substances that may be potentially harmful. Small objects can be inhaled into the respiratory tract, where it may cause a fatal obstruction of the airway. Other than this, the main risk for children is from poisoning.

Suspected poisoning is a common reason for children to be taken to a hospital emergency department, and is usually the result of them accidentally eating or drinking something harmful. In older children, it may sometimes be deliberate self-harm.

Measures to reduce the likelihood of poisoning, such as the introduction of childproof containers for medicines and household cleaning products, have reduced the number of poisonings in Australia and New Zealand, highlighting that the most important element in the management of poisoning is prevention rather than cure.

TOXIC SUBSTANCES

Accidental swallowing of drugs and household fluids is most likely to occur when a child is two to three years old. The most common poisonous substances ingested are family medicines and household products such as bleach and other cleaning products.

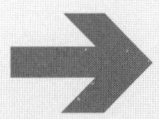

CHILDPROOF CAUTION
About one in five children under the age of five years are able to open childproof containers. Whether they have childproof lids or not, keep all dangerous substances out of reach of children.

Most poisonings do not result in major problems – eight out of ten accidental poisonings cause no harm, and most of the rest cause mild symptoms only. Fatalities are extremely rare – about one in 10 000 incidents. Occasionally, serious side effects do occur, most commonly from carbon monoxide fumes given off by fires (see page 212).

Toxicity of common medicines, products and plants

TOXICITY	MEDICINES	HOUSEHOLD PRODUCTS	PLANTS
Low	Contraceptive pill Antibiotics	Chalk, crayons Washing powder	Frangipani Eucalyptus
Medium	Paracetamol Salbutamol (Ventolin)	Bleach Disinfectants Window cleaners	Cacti Lantana Chilli plants
High	Alcoholic drinks Digoxin Iron Salicylate (aspirin) Tricyclic anti- depressants	Acids and alkalis Petroleum distillates Organophos- phate insecti- cides	Oleander (yellow) Deadly nightshade Compost and fertilisers

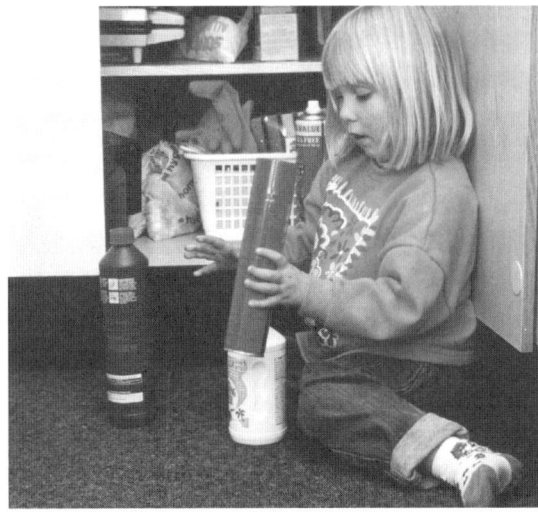

Make sure that cleaning products, which often contain poisonous substances, are kept in a cupboard secured with a childproof lock.

Medications that can cause serious problems include:

- aspirin
- paracetamol
- adult heart condition medicines, such as digoxin or betablockers
- iron supplement tablets
- tricyclic anti-depressants.

Symptoms of poisoning

Symptoms can vary enormously, from none at all to coma and death. Between these extremes are a variety of symptoms, including nausea and vomiting, abdominal pain, dizziness, headache, fever, lethargy and seizures. These symptoms are non-specific (meaning that any number of poisons can have the same initial symptoms), but should alert you to the possibility of accidental poisoning, particularly if no other cause is found. More usually, though, you will know if your child has put something in their mouth and what it was by the container.

If there is any doubt about the danger posed by something ingested, contact your GP or emergency department for advice. They will have information on drugs, household substances and common plants and fungi (mushrooms and toadstools) that may have been ingested.

FOREIGN BODIES

Another common problem, particularly with young children, is when they ingest small solid objects such as coins, marbles and small toys. These are collectively known in medicine as 'foreign bodies'.

Most of these objects will pass through the body unchanged and rarely cause problems, but occasionally they get stuck. The majority of foreign bodies are swallowed and therefore, if they do get stuck, it is likely to be at the end of the gullet (or oesophagus) at its junction with the stomach.

There is no point in looking for the foreign body in the child's nappy or faeces – this is unpleasant for you and will only cause you to worry unnecessarily if you don't find the object. Once foreign bodies have reached the stomach, they have passed the narrowest part of the

If a child has swallowed a foreign body, such as a coin or small toy, it will usually pass through the body, but may get stuck where the oesophagus joins the stomach.

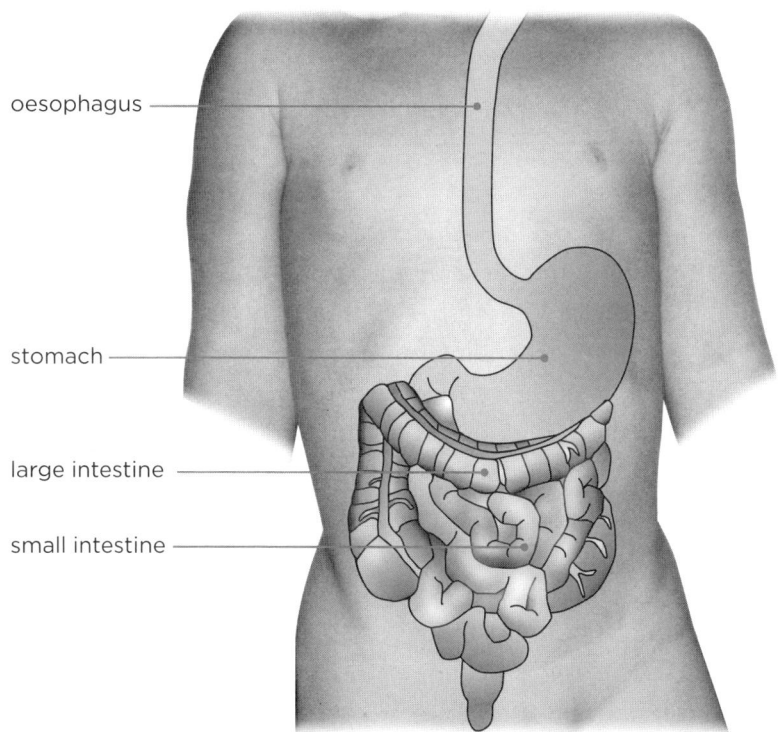

oesophagus

stomach

large intestine

small intestine

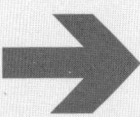

DANGER SIGNS

If your child swallows a small round battery ('button battery') – or puts a button battery up their nose – seek immediate medical assistance. These batteries can leak acid and erode the lining of the stomach or intestines and must be removed as soon as possible.

digestive tract and will carry on all the way through without any further difficulty. However, should your child have any abdominal pain, nausea or vomiting, it is wise to seek advice from your GP or emergency department.

Occasionally, small objects are inhaled and can lodge in the airways and lungs (trachea or bronchi). This may result in either partial or total blockage (obstruction) of the airway.

Any airway obstruction is an emergency and needs to be assessed and treated immediately. After swallowing a foreign body, if a child has any problems, such as noisy breathing or chest discomfort, they should be taken to the nearest emergency department.

At the doctor's

If your child looks very unwell, has taken dangerous substances or is not fully conscious, they will be given priority and seen quickly. If they look well and are not distressed, they may have to wait a while before they are seen, depending on the number and severity of illness of other patients waiting for medical care.

To help medical staff diagnose and judge the severity of the problem, give a clear and concise history. Certain information about possible ingestion of potentially harmful substances is required.

- What has been taken?
- How much has been taken?
- At what time did this occur?
- How did it occur?

If possible, take a sample of the substance or plant ingested (and its bottle or packet if there is one) to the hospital. This is very helpful to medical staff in identifying the toxin involved and the treatment.

Your child will be examined and have some observations performed, usually pulse and respiratory rate and oxygen levels via a small probe on their finger or foot. Other investigations may be necessary – including urine tests (to rule out urinary tract infections), blood tests (to look at the salts and signs of infection in the blood) or a chest x-ray. Rarely, other tests such as a CT scan of the head are carried out. After the tests the medical staff will decide if your child can go home or if they need to be admitted to the hospital for further assessment.

INFORMATION ABOUT POISONS
Poisons Information Centre Australia: 13 11 26
Poisons Information Centre New Zealand: 0800 764 766

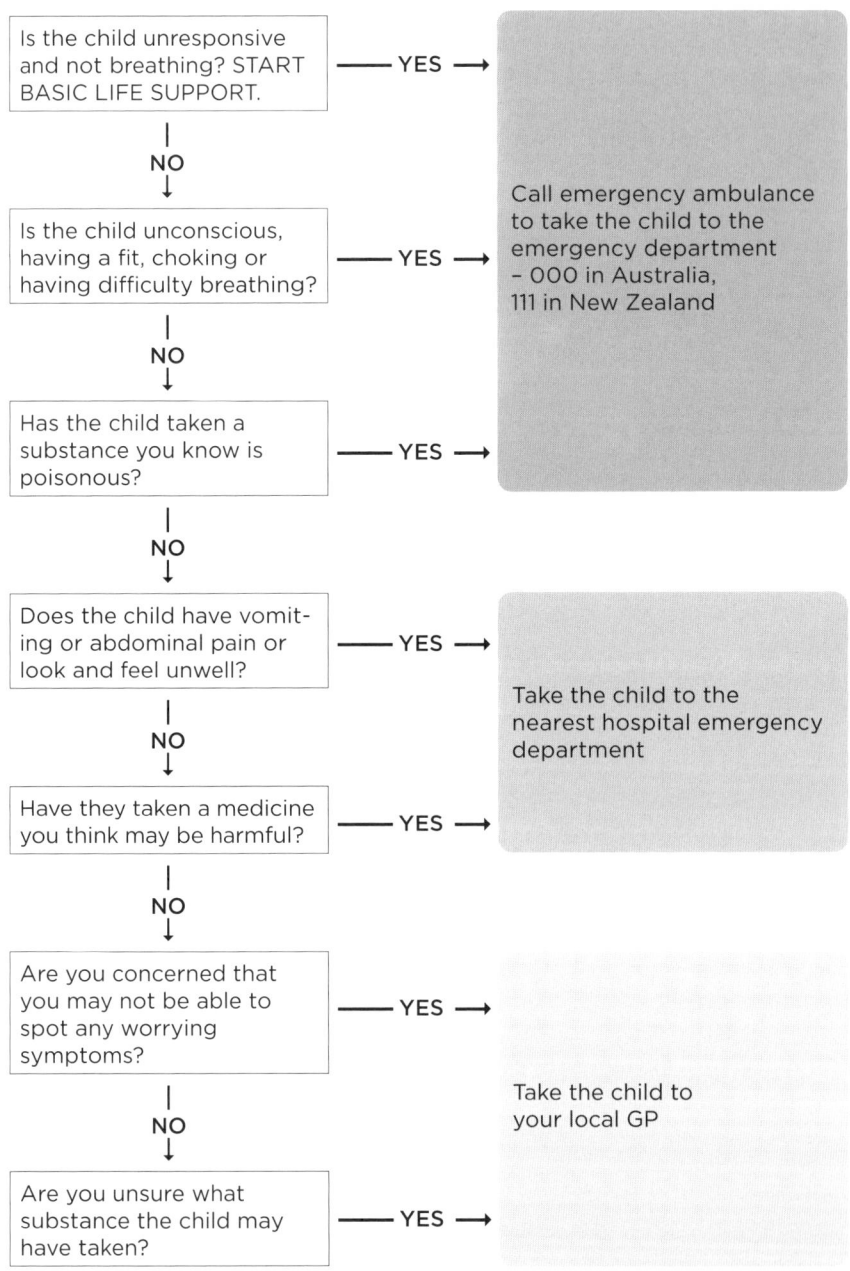

Is the child unresponsive and not breathing? START BASIC LIFE SUPPORT. —— YES →

NO ↓

Is the child unconscious, having a fit, choking or having difficulty breathing? —— YES →

NO ↓

Has the child taken a substance you know is poisonous? —— YES →

Call emergency ambulance to take the child to the emergency department – 000 in Australia, 111 in New Zealand

NO ↓

Does the child have vomiting or abdominal pain or look and feel unwell? —— YES →

NO ↓

Have they taken a medicine you think may be harmful? —— YES →

Take the child to the nearest hospital emergency department

NO ↓

Are you concerned that you may not be able to spot any worrying symptoms? —— YES →

NO ↓

Are you unsure what substance the child may have taken? —— YES →

Take the child to your local GP

21

BITES
AND STINGS

Australia has many spiders, snakes and marine creatures that can create serious medical problems if they bite or sting children. New Zealand has only one poisonous spider.

Most injuries are minor and will cause few serious problems, but sometimes severe illness can occur. It is important to know which dangerous creatures to watch out for and what immediate first aid measures are needed to deal with them.

From an early age children should be taught that some spiders and snakes are dangerous creatures and can even kill. Teach them not to approach, touch or tease spiders or snakes – or, in fact, any wild animal.

Dangerous spiders and snakes are usually found in natural bush environments, but occasionally in gardens, in public spaces such as parks, and sometimes even in and around the home. While contact with these creatures is not common, many children each year are taken to hospital for treatment after a bite or sting.

COMMON INSECT BITES AND STINGS

The price to pay for living in a warm, sometimes damp, environment is the presence of insects that may bite or sting. The results are mostly irritation and annoyance, and for most of Australia and New Zealand there are no significant parasites transmitted by these bites, although there are a few exceptions.

Mosquito bites

Mosquitoes are common but rarely carry serious diseases. Their bite mainly causes an irritating reaction at the site. However, in far north Queensland there have been cases of malaria caused by mosquitoes.

Mosquitoes breed in still water and these are the areas that will contain the highest concentration. If mosquitoes are a problem in your garden, look around for sources, such as still water in pots and ponds, and tip them out or dry them up if possible. Most mosquitoes are active at dawn and dusk, so this is when you need to be most careful. To prevent them biting your children, it is important they wear long sleeves and trousers and light-coloured clothing at these times because mosquitoes are attracted to darker colours (it gives them a degree of camouflage). Use insect repellent on exposed skin. The most effective repellents are those containing at least 10 per cent of a chemical called DEET. There is also some recent evidence that repellents containing lemon eucalyptus oil and, to a lesser degree, citronella have some mosquito-repellent properties.

TREATMENT

Most mosquito bites cause a small itchy lump that settles in approximately 48 hours. Some bites can cause larger and more painful swelling and these are best treated with painkillers, ice packs (wrapped in a towel) and antihistamine tablets or creams. Scratching mosquito bites, however tempting and satisfying, can lead to abrasions (open skin wounds) and infections. Teach your children not to do this.

Bee and wasp stings

Stings from bees or wasps can cause a painful, itchy lump at the site of the wound. Bee stings tend to be more painful than those of wasps and often the stinger is left behind by the bee. If this is the case, it should be removed by scraping it with a sharp object (such as a knife) rather than pulling it out. Pulling it can cause more venom to be released and a more painful reaction. Wasps do not leave a stinger behind. Bees will only sting once, whereas wasps can sting a person multiple times.

TREATMENT

For bee or wasp stings, relieve the pain with painkillers and apply an ice pack (wrapped in a towel) to the affected area. If you are concerned that your child is having a serious reaction to a sting, then call an ambulance – 000 in Australia, 111 in New Zealand.

Some people do have severe allergic reactions to bees and wasps, although this is not common. If a child has a history of severe allergy then they are often prescribed an adrenaline syringe, called an EpiPen. If a child who has this history and is carrying an EpiPen gets stung, use this urgently, according to instructions (which are found on the device). As a rule of thumb, if a child appears unwell after a sting and is known to be allergic, you should definitely use the EpiPen. The use of this device is extremely unlikely to cause any medical problems, but in a very allergic child it will be life saving.

SPIDERS

There are approximately 2900 species of spiders in Australia. Of these, only a few are known to be dangerous. A bite from a red-back or funnel-web spider, or the closely related mouse spider, can cause death. Many other spiders can cause pain and swelling at the site of a bite, but these often need little treatment. For the majority of spider bites the only treatment necessary is pain relief – for example, with paracetamol or ibuprofen.

SEVERE SYMPTOMS OF SPIDER BITES
- Pain at the site of the bite
- Sweating, which may only be present in the bitten area
- Vomiting.

Red-back spider

The red-back spider has a wide distribution throughout Australia and can be found in and around homes and gardens. They are distinctive because of the recognisable red marking on their backs. These spiders should not be approached at any time. The females are larger and more dangerous than the males, but will only become aggressive and bite if threatened. Most bites – about four out of five – do not result in any symptoms other than pain and swelling at the site of the bite.

Severe symptoms following a red-back spider bite are:

- pain at the bite site
- sweating (which may only be present in the bitten area)
- vomiting.

Take a child with these severe symptoms to an emergency department.

If the child is exhibiting local pain only and that pain increases one to two hours after the bite despite adequate pain relief (paracetamol or ibuprofen), they should also be taken to the emergency department.

TREATMENT

For first aid treatment of a red-back spider bite:

- assess your child's airways, breathing and circulation
- provide pain relief in the form of paracetamol or ibuprofen
- apply an ice pack to the affected arm or leg – do not put the ice directly on the skin, but wrap it in a cloth
- elevate the affected arm or leg
- take your child to the nearest emergency department if they are exhibiting severe symptoms (see above).

A compression immobilisation bandage (see box, page 227) is not recommended for these bites because this can increase the pain to the bitten area.

In the emergency department, doctors may need to give the child the specific red-back spider antivenom to neutralise the toxins from the spider bite. This antivenom is given by injection into a muscle.

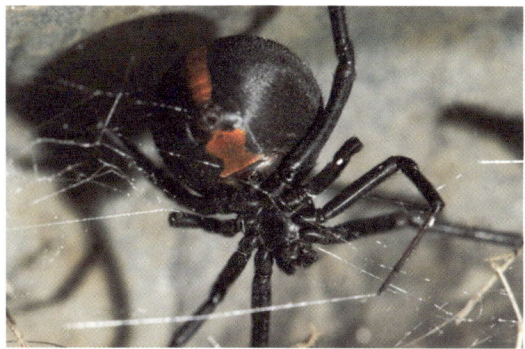

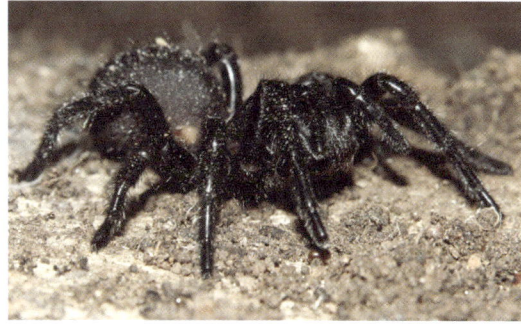

The bite of the red-back spider (above) can cause severe symptoms. The Sydney funnel-web spider (left) is one of the most dangerous spiders in the world.

Katipo spider

This is the only poisonous spider in New Zealand. It is related to the red-back spider, although it is not as venomous. It is small to medium sized and has a black body with an irregular white-bordered red stripe on its back.

TREATMENT

For severe symptoms – which are similar to those for the red-back spider – take the child to the nearest emergency department, where antivenom may be administered. First aid treatments for bites from the katipo spider are the same as for the red-back.

Funnel-web spider

The funnel-web spider is one of the most dangerous spiders in the world. They are big, black, hairy, with large fangs and are very aggressive. The male spider is more dangerous than the female, and is more likely to be encountered due to its habit of night-time wandering in search of the female's burrow. There are over 40 species of funnel-web spider, but the Sydney funnel-web spider is the only one that is known to be lethal. Sydney funnel-web spiders have also been known to enter houses, particularly in wet weather.

The majority of bites from funnel-webs do not result in any symptoms other than local pain and swelling at the site of the bite. However, about 10 to 25 per cent of them will cause severe symptoms that need treatment in a hospital's emergency department.

A single bite from a Sydney funnel-web spider can be potentially lethal in less than an hour. The bite is immediately painful. Other symptoms that may develop are:

- abdominal pain
- sweating
- vomiting
- headache
- dizziness.

TREATMENT

First aid treatment includes: providing pain relief in the form of paracetamol or ibuprofen, and compression immobilisation bandaging (see the box opposite). If your child becomes unconscious, then a systematic approach to assessing them should be made.

- assess and check the airways, breathing and circulation
- provide pain relief
- apply compression immobilisation bandaging
- take them to an emergency department.

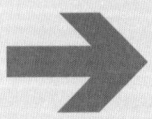

CAUTION
With all spider bites, do **not** attempt to capture the spider – this may result in further bites. Multiple bites can cause severe symptoms.

COMPRESSION IMMOBILISATION BANDAGING

Compression immobilisation bandaging (CIB) can be life saving because it prevents venom from a bite travelling in the blood-stream, thus allowing time for the victim to be taken to hospital and given an antivenom injection.

CIB is performed by applying a bandage (preferably a crepe one), starting from the foot or hand of the affected limb and working towards the body.

If a bandage is not available you can use a pair of tights or some ripped up pieces of clothing torn into strips about 7 to 10 centimetres wide. The bandage should be applied firmly, but not so tightly that it causes any discomfort.

Once the bandage has been applied, the affected limb should be immobilised to restrict its movement (movement may cause the venom to spread into the bloodstream more quickly). Ideally, the child should not be moved. Call for an ambulance to take them to the nearest hospital emergency department.

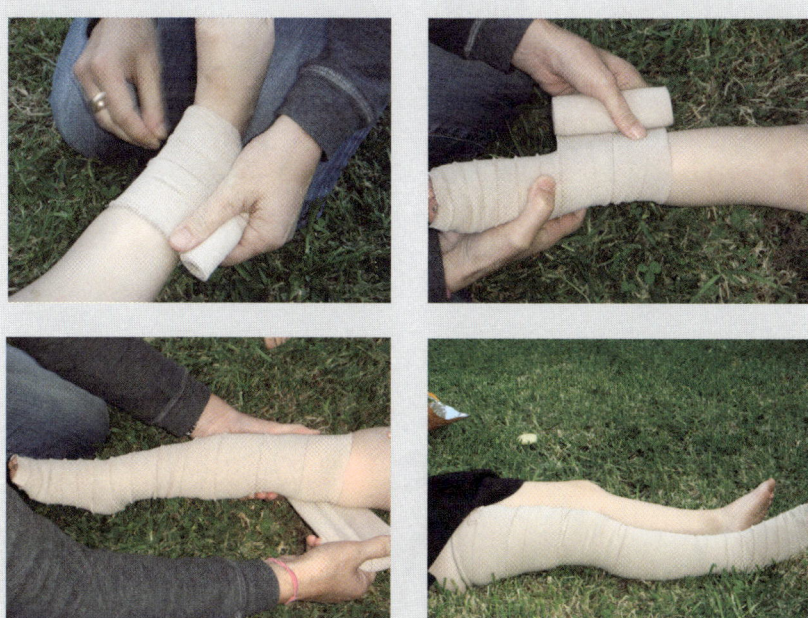

Mouse spiders

These spiders have a widespread distribution in Australia, and are often found in swimming pools and gardens. They look similar to funnel-webs, being medium to large, bulbous and mostly black. Less than 10 per cent of mouse spider bites contain venom, and most bites cause little or no symptoms. Occasionally significant symptoms appear, similar to those caused by the venom of a funnel-web spider.

TREATMENT

Treat as for funnel-web bites. The venom from mouse spiders responds to funnel-web spider antivenom.

Huntsman spiders

Huntsman spiders are fairly large hairy spiders with long legs. They are often found around the house. In fact, they are a relatively harmless group of spiders. They usually only bite if threatened so, as with all spiders, teach your child not to touch or tease them.

TREATMENT

Their bites cause local pain and swelling only and should be treated with analgesia and ice, and ask for advice from your GP. If this does not work, or if the spider is not clearly identified, seek urgent help by taking the child to the nearest emergency department.

Other spiders

If your child has been bitten by any other spider, or if you could not identify the spider, you should:

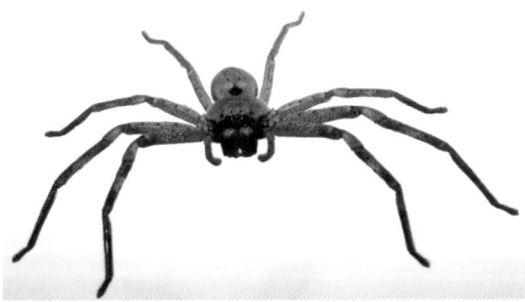

Huntsman spiders are large and hairy.

- assess their airways, breathing and circulation if they are unconscious or not breathing normally
- if there is pain, provide paracetamol or ibuprofen
- apply compression immobilisation bandaging
- apply an ice pack to reduce the local pain and swelling – if the pain does not respond to this, take the child to the nearest emergency department
- take them to an emergency department if the child complains of nausea, headache or dizziness, or is sweating or vomiting.

SNAKES

New Zealand has no snakes, but there are 75 species in Australia. Fifty-five of these are venomous, so there are many capable of biting a child and injecting lethal venom. Between 1000 and 3000 snake bites are reported in Australia each year and cause one to four deaths. Brown snake bites kill more than any other species. Other potentially lethal snakes include tiger snakes, taipans and red–bellied black snakes.

However, over 90 per cent of the time snake bites contain no venom and cause local pain and anxiety only. If venom has spread into the bloodstream, potential symptoms that may occur include:

- abdominal pain and vomiting
- headache and dizziness
- difficulty speaking and breathing
- confusion and decreased or loss of consciousness
- weakness.

TREATMENT

All snake bites can be managed in the same way. The first aid treatment of snake bites includes:

- pain relief (paracetamol or ibuprofen)
- compression immobilisation bandaging (see page 227), which prevents the venom from travelling through the bloodstream, allowing time for the child to be taken to hospital, where they will be given an antivenom injection.

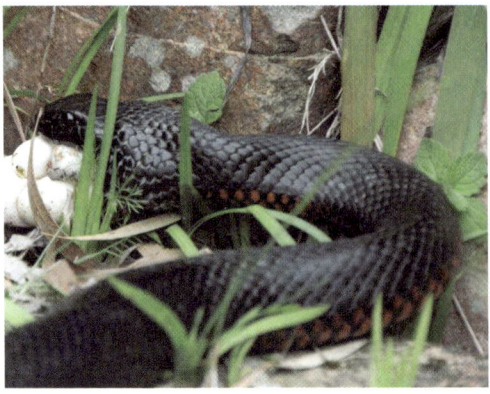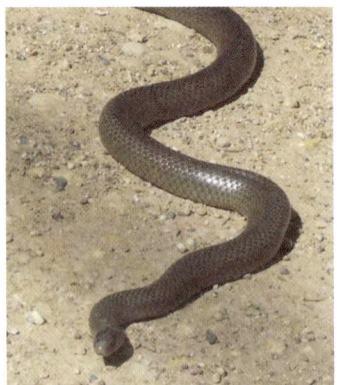

Among the most venomous snakes found in Australia are the red-bellied black snake (left) and the brown snake (right).

You should not wash or suck the wound. Do not throw away any clothes you may have removed from the child because these can often be used by medical staff to identify the venom (if it has contaminated the cloth). As in the case of spider bites, antivenom by injection may be needed for severe snake bites.

If your child becomes unconscious or has difficulty breathing:

- check their airways, breathing and circulation
- provide pain relief
- apply compression immobilisation bandaging
- take them to an emergency department or call 000.

MARINE CREATURES

In Australian waters, jellyfish are responsible for the majority of stings from marine life. Most of these only cause pain and swelling at the site of the sting, but in some instances this can be deadly. Stings occur when jellyfish tentacles touch the skin and venom is injected, which causes an immediate sharp pain at the point of contact.

There are two jellyfish in Australian waters that can be deadly and both are found in the tropical sea waters off the coasts of northern Queensland, the Northern Territory and the north of Western

Australia. These are the box jellyfish and the irukandji jellyfish. The waters of Australia also contain one venomous octopus species: the blue-ringed octopus.

Box jellyfish

These are one of the most venomous sea creatures in the world. They are pale blue and transparent-like, with a box-like cube and tentacles that grow up to 15 centimetres long.

The sting of a box jellyfish can be fatal in less than a minute. However, the majority of these stings do not result in venom being injected into the body, but they cause local pain and swelling. Other symptoms are:

- difficulty breathing
- abdominal pain
- sweating
- vomiting
- headache
- dizziness.

TREATMENT

If a child shows any signs of difficulty with breathing, speaking or moving, they should be taken immediately to the nearest emergency department. This is the only jellyfish for which there is an antivenom and this may be life saving if given early enough. If the affected child is not breathing you should perform basic life support (see Chapter 24). Otherwise, assess their airways, breathing and circulation and get medical assistance.

For minor stings provide pain relief, apply an ice pack (ensuring you wrap it in a towel first so it doesn't have direct contact with the skin) and wash the site with tolerably hot water (not vinegar, as suggested for other jellyfish, below).

Irukandji jellyfish

These are a family of small jellyfish (about 1 centimetre long). They mostly cause minor symptoms after a sting, but sometimes there might be abdominal pain, vomiting, sweating, headache, dizziness and difficulty breathing. There have been reports of death following irukandji stings. The treatment for these stings is the same as for box jellyfish stings. There is no antivenom.

Other jellyfish

Most jellyfish stings are harmless. The pain from the local venom sting is usually short-lasting and not severe.

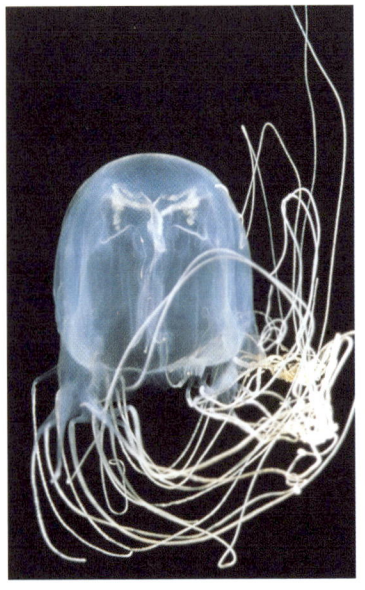

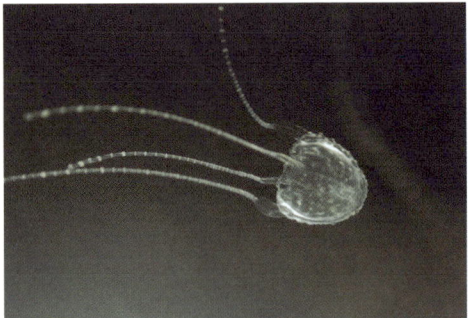

The box jellyfish (left) and the irukandji jellyfish (above).

Below: *The common bluebottle (left) and the blue-ringed octopus (right).*

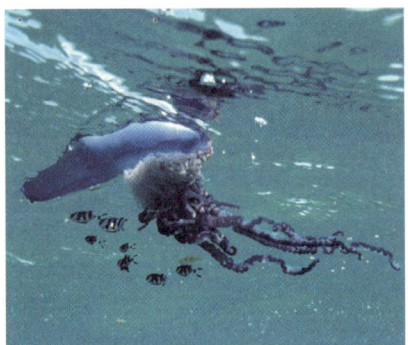

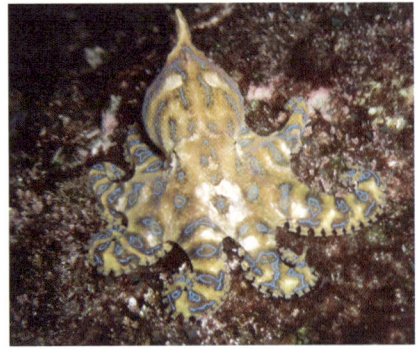

TREATMENT

For most jellyfish stings, rinse the affected part of the body in sea water – rinsing in fresh water may cause more venom to be released from small parts of tentacles still attached to the skin. If there are any visible tentacles on the skin, these should be removed using tweezers or a gloved hand.

For stings from the common bluebottle, standing under a hot shower for 20 minutes can ease the pain. Otherwise apply tolerably hot water to the affected part, being careful not to scald the area. Vinegar has been shown to reduce firing of the parts of the jellyfish that contain the toxins and to reduce the pain from jellyfish stings. This should be applied to the affected area if no hot water is available.

In summary, treat most jellyfish stings by:

- rinsing the affected area in sea water
- removing any tentacles
- washing in tolerably hot water or in vinegar if no water is available
- standing under a hot shower for 20 minutes if stung by a bluebottle jellyfish
- providing pain relief.

Blue-ringed octopus

These are four species of similar octopuses, each about the size of a golf ball with venom capable of killing a human. They are fairly common down the east coast of Australia, from far north Queensland to the southern New South Wales coast. They have characteristic blue and black rings on their bodies.

Most stings from these octopuses cause only local pain and swelling; rarely, more generalised symptoms, such as vomiting, breathing difficulties, collapse or sudden death, may occur.

TREATMENT

There is no known antidote to blue-ringed octopus stings. If you suspect your child has been stung by one of these, call an ambulance to take them to the nearest emergency department.

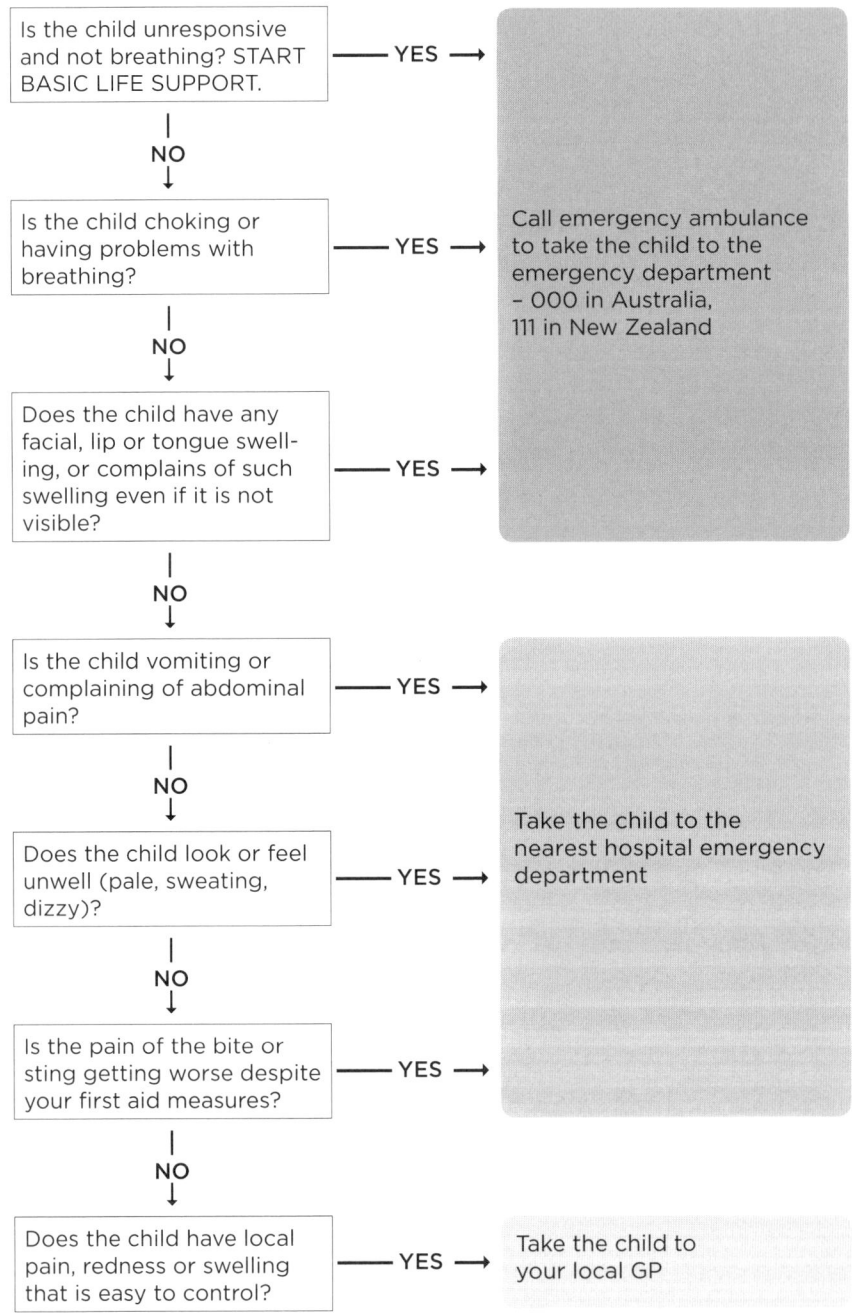

Is the child unresponsive and not breathing? START BASIC LIFE SUPPORT. ——YES——→

NO ↓

Is the child choking or having problems with breathing? ——YES——→ Call emergency ambulance to take the child to the emergency department – 000 in Australia, 111 in New Zealand

NO ↓

Does the child have any facial, lip or tongue swelling, or complains of such swelling even if it is not visible? ——YES——→

NO ↓

Is the child vomiting or complaining of abdominal pain? ——YES——→

NO ↓

Does the child look or feel unwell (pale, sweating, dizzy)? ——YES——→ Take the child to the nearest hospital emergency department

NO ↓

Is the pain of the bite or sting getting worse despite your first aid measures? ——YES——→

NO ↓

Does the child have local pain, redness or swelling that is easy to control? ——YES——→ Take the child to your local GP

22

DROWNING, HYPOTHERMIA AND ELECTRICAL INJURIES

A child who nearly drowns or suffers from hypothermia or an electrical injury should be administered emergency first aid. Your child may have a cardiac arrest due to one of these environmental injuries, so you need to know how to handle that situation.

As with other injuries, the best approach is to check airways, breathing and circulation (see page 252) and provide basic life support (see Chapter 24). You must always follow the systematic approach of assessment so that nothing is missed – for instance, a spinal injury resulting from a fall in shallow water, or hypothermia occurring in a child who has nearly drowned.

DROWNING

Drowning is a leading cause of death in children in Australia and New Zealand and preventative measures should always be taken to minimise the risks of children being left unsupervised near bodies of water (see Chapter 17: Injury prevention).

REMEMBER YOUR ABC

Airway
- open the child's airway to see if they are breathing
- use the head tilt, chin lift technique (but not if head or neck injuries are suspected)
- remember the jaw thrust technique in trauma.

Breathing
- look, listen and feel to see if the child is breathing
- if the child is not breathing, start mouth-to-mouth resuscitation.

Circulation
- check to see if the child has a pulse
- if there is no pulse, start chest compressions.

These water areas include the ocean, rivers and lakes, smaller streams and canals, swimming pools and even garden ponds. Tragic incidents can also occur in the most innocuous of circumstances and careful supervision of children in the bath, for example, is essential if drowning is to be prevented.

On average, 35 children die each year from drowning in Australia; in New Zealand drowning is over twice the Australian rate per capita, at 20 deaths per year. In 2006–07 the most common place of drowning for children was in domestic swimming pools, with the second most frequent location being the bath. Deaths by drowning in lagoons and lakes dropped by 53 per cent over the previous five years, but those at the beach increased by 39 per cent. Boys over four years were almost three times as likely as girls to drown.

Drowning occurs when water fills the lungs. If the lungs are full of water for a short period, a child initially will stop breathing and then will suffer a cardiac arrest caused by the lack of oxygen getting to the heart and brain. Death will occur unless steps are taken to stop and reverse the process.

TREATMENT

Starting basic life support (see Chapter 24) as early as possible greatly influences the chances of survival. You need to begin by calling for help (000, or 111 in New Zealand), then assess the child's airways, breathing and circulation (see page 252) and act accordingly. You may do this initial assessment while the child (and possibly you) is still in the water. It is imperative it is done as soon as possible.

Firstly, check that the airway is open. If not, use the head–tilt/chin–lift method (see page 254) unless you suspect head or neck injuries, which may occur, for instance, if the child has dived into shallow water. Then the neck should be supported and immobilised if possible and the airway should be opened using the jaw thrust manoeuvre (see page 255). Although maintaining neck immobilisation protects the spine from injury, this should not take priority over opening the airway. If the airway is not opened everything else will fail.

If the child is breathing, they should be removed from the water, placed in the recovery position (see page 262) and observed until help arrives. When moving a child from the water, take particular care that the position of their body remains horizontal if possible by lifting their legs at the same time as the torso.

If there is no evidence of breathing, assisted breaths (mouth to mouth) should be given as soon as possible. This may need to be done while the child is still in the water or, if this is not possible, immediately after they have been removed from the water.

The pulse should then be assessed. This is a skill that some health professionals find difficult in emergency situations, but you should attempt to look for signs, or lack, of circulation. In cardiac arrest there are no spontaneous breaths, no coughing or gagging and no spontaneous movement. If these are absent and you cannot feel any pulse, chest compressions should be started. It is not possible to do this effectively while the child is still in the water – they must be removed to a flat, hard surface first.

If there is a pulse but no breathing, rescue breathing should be continued until there is a change in the child's condition or until the emergency services arrive, while periodically (every minute) monitoring to make sure that there is still a pulse present.

The SAFE approach (see Chapter 23) should always be followed so that rescuers do not put themselves at risk. It is much more difficult for emergency services to co-ordinate the rescue and resuscitation of multiple casualties (the child and their rescuers, for instance) than that of a single patient. If you have assessed that the child is breathing and has a pulse, keep them still and warm, in a safe place away from danger, and keep checking both their breathing and pulse.

HANDING OVER TO MEDICAL PERSONNEL

A child who has recovered from a near-drowning incident needs to be seen by a doctor and will always need to be admitted to hospital for a period of observation. When handing over their care to a doctor or a member of the emergency services it is important to provide the following information, which may subsequently be of use.

- Was the episode witnessed?
- Does the child have any history of trauma or epilepsy?
- How long was the child submerged in the water?
- How long before basic life support was commenced?

HYPOTHERMIA

This is when body temperature drops below 35°C. Normal body temperature is 36.5°C (or 97.7°F). Hypothermia is caused by exposure to the cold and is often associated with episodes of near drowning. It should always be considered in these circumstances. It may also occur for a variety of other reasons, such as prolonged exposure to the elements outdoors. Even indoors the very young, like the elderly, are at risk of hypothermia if their environment is not adequately heated.

Those at the extremes of age are more at risk of hypothermia because their mechanisms for controlling their internal temperature may not be able to cope with even relatively minor changes in the environment. Added to this, they are often not mobile and independent and therefore cannot move themselves out of a cold atmosphere or put on warm clothes to prevent cooling. The very young should never be exposed to the extremes of cold if possible; however, if exposed to cold conditions, they should be kept warm and covered, especially their heads from which there is a large heat loss in babies, infants and young children.

The first symptom of hypothermia is shivering, which is the body's natural response to cold, and this occurs as the body attempts to produce heat by small contractions of muscles. Young infants do not have this shivering reflex and therefore cannot protect themselves against the cold as well as older children can. If the child gets any colder there may be confusion or disorientation, followed by a reduction in their level of consciousness, ending in coma, or unconsciousness. When the body temperature gets as low as this, their heart may suffer problems with rhythm and may stop altogether.

In these circumstances, even though the heart has stopped, there is still a possibility of good recovery if basic life support (see Chapter 24) is initiated and continued while the child is warmed. This is because the vital organs – such as the brain, heart and kidneys – are cooled to such an extent that metabolism slows and the requirement for oxygen drops. This means they will survive longer than normal, even if there is a poor supply of blood and therefore a poor supply of oxygen.

TREATMENT
- If the child is unconscious, the airway should be assessed and opened if necessary.
- If there is no breathing, assisted breathing should be started immediately.
- The pulse should be checked and chest compressions started if there is no pulse.

In a hypothermic child, basic life support may have to be continued for a considerable time while they are warmed. This is because the heart will not properly recover until the body temperature rises above a certain level.

It is imperative that you call for emergency medical help – 000 in Australia, 111 in New Zealand – and the child is transferred to a hospital by ambulance as soon as possible. Staff at an emergency department have other methods for warming patients, such as breathing warm air into the lungs and infusing warm fluids into the veins and stomach.

Basic life support should not be interrupted during this transfer – it should not be stopped until the child has reached hospital. The golden rule in treating hypothermic children is that there is always a chance of survival, even after prolonged periods of being cold and without a pulse.

If the child is conscious but cold and shivering, their cold or wet clothing should be removed and they should be warmed with warm, dry blankets or towels. A warm bath (at a temperature that is comfortable to the touch without causing burning or scalding to the skin) may also help warm up the child. If they are drowsy then a bath should not be used; instead, they should be warmed using dry blankets in warm surroundings.

ELECTRICAL INJURIES

Electric shock is any injury that results from electricity. Electrocution is death due to an electric shock. Children account for about a third of all patients with electrical injuries, a small proportion of which are fatal.

Electrical injuries range from minor shocks from isolated sources such as batteries to large and devastating lightning strikes, which result in a huge electric shock across the heart and may cause cardiac arrest. The most common electrical injury in children, however, is from the electricity mains supply in homes.

With electrical injuries, make sure the patient is not connected to any electrical source before assessment or treatment is attempted. For *safety*, the power needs to be switched off at the mains. The rescuer's

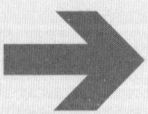

CAUTION
No attempt should be made to touch a child or pull them away from the source of an electrical accident until the electricity supply has been turned off.

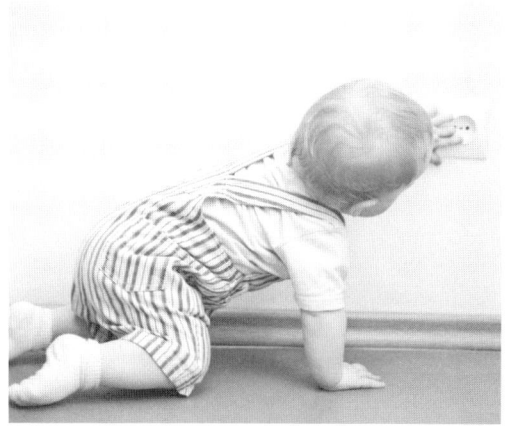

Electric sockets within reach of young children should be fitted with covers.

safety in this instance, as always, is paramount. There is no point attempting to rescue a child if you also become a victim. This does not save the child and will create another victim who needs help.

TREATMENT

Always approach the child using the SAFE method (see Chapter 23). A systematic assessment of airways, breathing and circulation (see page 252) is important if other problems are not to be missed; for example, injuries resulting from being thrown from the electric source. If the child is unconscious you should assume they have a neck injury and support and immobilise their neck during the assessment and treatment (see page 253).

If there appears to be only minor injuries or burns the child should still be assessed either by your GP or in an emergency department, as even seemingly superficial burns can actually be quite deep and may need significant intervention and treatment.

PART IV

ESSENTIALS

You need to know the essentials of caring for a seriously ill or injured child. The backbone of any first aid or emergency life-saving action is safety and knowing how to perform basic life support. When you hand the sick child over to the medical professionals it is helpful if you can tell them the things they need to know and how you can give this information succinctly.

Before rushing to the aid of others, you need to consider your own safety. This is often difficult because your focus will be on your child. But if you get injured in the process of helping them you may not be able to assist them as you would wish, and you may also become a casualty who needs to be cared for. In this way, you distract or divide the help of others because they need to assist you as well your child. This is what the SAFE approach to dealing with emergencies is all about.

Many severe childhood illnesses and injuries either respond promptly or are prevented from getting worse by a few simple actions – such as placing the child in the recovery position. Having a working knowledge of basic life support does save lives. The principles are simple and these very basic interventions may prove essential in an emergency.

In previous chapters we stressed the importance of when to get help for your child, from your GP, the nearest emergency department or by calling an ambulance. But your involvement does not stop when you take your child to a healthcare professional. It is important you know what to expect next, to have an idea of what is involved when you hand over their care to the professionals. You will be more help to your child if you are able to communicate the problem by being aware of what the healthcare professionals need to know, and what the doctors or other medical staff will do to assist them to recovery.

Knowing what to do for a seriously ill or injured child can make a huge difference. It will give you the ability to potentially save your child's life.

23

THE 'SAFE' APPROACH

When your child is injured or ill it immediately makes you want to rush in and help. This will be your first reaction.

However, it is important to be aware of your surroundings and any possible dangers you may encounter, or indeed create, before starting to administer aid.

When approaching a potential casualty, your first priority should be your own safety. This might sound selfish or callous, but think about it: if you enter a dangerous or contaminated environment without thought or preparation, the chances are that you too may become a casualty. If this happens, it could mean:

- a delay in life-saving treatment for the child because you need treatment too
- a delay in rescuing the child because you will need rescuing also
- the need for more rescuers to help you as well.

This not only means you have exposed yourself to the possibility of injury, illness or death, it means that you may have prevented your child from getting the opportunity to have the necessary and immediate first aid they need.

ASSESSING THE SITUATION AND THE CHILD

To avoid danger to yourself, a safe, structured approach is necessary:

- **S** - **s**hout for help
- **A** - **a**pproach with care
- **F** - **f**ree from danger
- **E** - **e**valuate airways, breathing and circulation.

Shout for help

Any situation where there is an ill or injured child is stressful, demanding and potentially urgent. This means the last thing that you want or need is to be dealing with it on your own. This is true of healthcare professionals as much as anyone else, which is why they are taught to shout loudly for help as soon as they recognise a problem and to continue shouting until help arrives.

If there are bystanders with mobile phones, shout to them to dial 000 (or 111 in New Zealand) while you are assessing the situation and/or attempting to treat your child. Shouting can also mean calling for an ambulance as well as yelling to other people to keep them at a safe distance until a trained professional has had a chance to assess the situation and treat the child.

Approach with care

Some hazards such as live electricity are obvious dangers, but people's desire to help is sometimes so strong that safety needs – such as disconnecting the electricity supply – can get forgotten in the heat of the moment.

A careful approach means you evaluate the situation before you go to the injured or ill child to ensure you don't put yourself in harm's way. Although this is most obvious in trauma involving hazardous situations, such as car accidents where the vehicle is in danger of igniting, it is useful to remember in any situation. Always approach a situation with care and assess any potential dangers before you step in.

Free from danger

This means that, having assessed the scene and ensured that you will not become another victim, you either remove the cause of the injury from the child or remove the child from the cause of injury to prevent harm continuing. To use the electricity example, it is pointless trying to resuscitate an electric shock victim if the electric shock is continuing.

Evaluate ABC

This is discussed and explored in more detail in Chapter 24 on basic life support, but essentially the assessment and treatment of an ill or injured child needs to be done in a systematic way to ensure nothing is missed and that potentially serious problems, those that are the greatest threat to life and will cause harm the fastest, are assessed and treated in the correct order. This takes the form of checking the child's:

- airway
- breathing
- circulation.

The ABC approach is extended further in some instances to include checking the child's:

- disability, or neurological status, particularly the level of consciousness, and pain relief
- exposure, environment (such as temperature) and everything else.

Remember, harm can be caused most quickly by obstruction of the airway, including the mouth, throat and windpipe; second, by being unable to breathe properly for reasons other than airway obstruction; third, by problems with circulation such as bleeding;

fourth, by problems with the brain and nerves which are not caused by ABC problems; and finally by environmental problems, such as low temperature, that affect the body.

When medical professionals use this order to assess how ill a child is they examine the airway visually, measure the breathing rate and any increased effort needed to breathe, measure the circulation by how fast the blood returns to an area when it is pressed and by taking the pulse if possible, gauge the level of consciousness by whether the child is alert, responding to voice or pain or is unresponsive, and then also examine them back and front, top to toe, to make sure there are not things missed on the first look such as a meningococcal rash or an injury that cannot be seen when they are completely dressed.

RISKS AND HAZARDS

Common hazards facing a potential rescuer are traffic, falling masonry and other objects, electricity, and fumes or smoke from a fire. These are often the things that have caused the illness or injury to the child in the first place. In many cases, a little commonsense can avoid serious complications. For example, if your child is involved in a motor vehicle accident, turning the engine off will interrupt the fuel supply and lessen the risk of an engine fire. It is important to stop, look and think for a few seconds before rushing in to the aid of the child.

You should also consider minimising risks to yourself and others. In a car accident, for example, you may be able to place your car in a safe position so that it acts as a warning for oncoming traffic and use hazard triangles or warning lights. In all instances, it is important to cooperate with and take advice from any emergency services.

If it is necessary and doesn't pose a risk to you, you can remove a child from a dangerous environment to a safe one before basic life support or first aid is carried out – for example, taking an unconscious child from a burning building. If trauma is suspected or witnessed, care should be taken to protect the child's neck and back to prevent causing or worsening a possible spinal injury. Their head and body should be held and turned as a unit, and should be supported to prevent rolling, twisting or tilting (see page 253).

If the problem involves an electricity supply, the current must be turned off at the mains before any attempt is made to move or aid the child. If you attempt to treat a case of electrocution without doing this you may very well be injured yourself, which means the chances of you being able to effectively treat the injured child have gone and you will also need to be treated, diverting resources from the child. Needless to say, there is a definite risk to your life if you ignore this advice as well as that of the child.

POTENTIAL FOR CROSS-INFECTION

Cross-infection is when an infection is passed from the child to the person giving medical aid – for example, during mouth-to-mouth resuscitation. However, the risk of cross-infection during basic life support procedures is extremely small, but there have been reports of isolated incidents involving the transmission of diseases such as herpes simplex (cold sores), salmonella (food poisoning) and meningitis. To put this in perspective, one study showed that over a 22-year period not a single case was reported among New York City firemen of an infectious disease being transmitted following mouth-to-mouth resuscitation.

People have recently been concerned about the transmission of HIV and hepatitis B during basic life support. Both these infections occur via bodily fluids, such as blood, semen and vaginal secretions. Saliva and vomit are not thought to be infectious unless there is a break in the skin or inside the mouth. As children have a lower incidence than adults of these serious infectious diseases, the chances of catching one while giving basic life support is even smaller.

Having said all that, it is sensible to adopt precautions when possible such as the use of breathing masks in mouth-to-mouth resuscitation, and gloves and eye protection if you have them handy, although this may not always be practicable outside a hospital environment.

24

BASIC LIFE SUPPORT

Successful basic life support (BLS) can save the life of a child in respiratory or cardiac arrest. BLS is a sequence of precisely timed life-saving manoeuvres that includes cardiopulmonary resuscitation (CPR, or mouth-to-mouth resuscitation) used in the assessment and treatment of a child needing immediate medical aid.

BLS maximises the chances of survival of children in medical need. The reasons they have cardiac arrest are generally because a severe illness has led to a lack of oxygen or fluids. This is potentially more likely to be reversible than any of the causes that lead to adults having a heart attack.

BLS can be performed by anyone who has the training. But research shows that poor teaching and a lack of regular practice can degrade BLS skills in a very short time. This illustrates the need for you to keep 'current' with your skills and knowledge to make sure that you will be able to act quickly and correctly in the rare instances they are required. Unfortunately, the number of people trained in

BLS in Australia and New Zealand is still low compared with other developed countries, especially the USA.

THEORY OF BLS

If a child has stopped breathing they have respiratory arrest. If they have stopped breathing and their heart has stopped beating, then they are in cardiorespiratory arrest (or cardiac arrest). The body needs oxygen to survive and the aim of BLS is to provide this oxygen to the vital organs (especially the heart and the brain) when normal breathing and blood flow have stopped.

To do this, first you must breathe for the child and then provide a 'pump' to get their blood around the body to the organs that need oxygen the most, such as the brain. By following some basic techniques, you can support life in an ill or injured child single-handedly until recovery occurs or help arrives.

The exact BLS techniques that need to be used depend on the size of the child, but the critical step in each technique is to deliver oxygen, and this must be your priority. Basic life support is based on the simple rule of ABC:

- **A** is for airway
- **B** is for breathing
- **C** is for circulation.

Why is it taught this way?

The best and most effective assessment and treatment should be carried out in this order of priority: first check airways, then breathing, then circulation. This ensures optimal care. The rationale is that a child will die first from a blocked airway, then from breathing problems, and then from problems with their circulation.

If there is a problem with the airway no oxygen is getting into the lungs, and therefore no matter how much the child tries to breathe or how much their heart pumps, no oxygen will get to the organs that need it. If they are not breathing then their blood will not have enough oxygen in it to support life, even if the heart is still pumping. Breathing is therefore the next priority after the airway is clear.

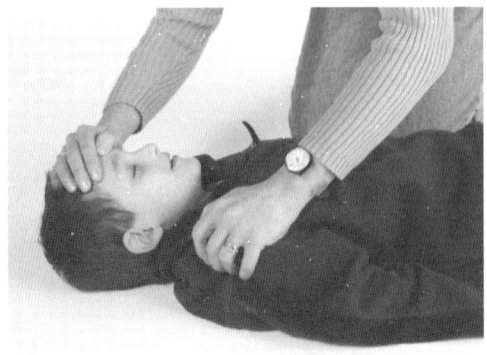

The first thing to do is assess just how responsive the child is.

This order of assessment and treatment is the backbone of BLS. That is why this approach is repeated throughout this book – it is the vital first step in providing your child with the best chance of survival.

INITIAL ASSESSMENT OF RESPONSIVENESS

When you approach an injured or ill child, you initially assess their responsiveness.

A simple 'Hello, are you all right?' with a gentle shake of the shoulders will suffice. If the child responds, a lot of meaningful information has been obtained. Firstly, the child's airway must be open, allowing air to come out from the lungs. Secondly, they must be breathing to enable them to speak. Thirdly, the child's circulation must be functioning because the brain is getting enough oxygen to perform the simple response of speaking. An awareness of the basic workings of the body, with an idea of what may go wrong, enables you to perform a rapid assessment in the same manner as a health professional.

In smaller children and infants a meaningful reply is unlikely to be forthcoming, but valuable information can still be gained. If the child opens their eyes, makes any purposeful movement or makes a sound to reply to someone's voice, then you can be assured their airway is open, they are breathing and their circulation is functioning.

In cases where trauma has occurred, such as a child being knocked down by a car, you must pay attention to their neck. They may have a cervical spine injury (see page 193). In practice, this means keeping the head and neck still and supported throughout resuscitation if possible, although this should not take priority over opening the airway. When approaching a child in this situation, place one of your hands on their forehead and use the other to gently shake their arm. They should not be moved unnecessarily as this may aggravate a possible injury.

If you are on your own and the child's heart has stopped beating and they have stopped breathing (cardiorespiratory arrest), it is recommended that one minute of basic life support (cardiopulmonary resuscitation or CPR) be administered before trying to get help (by calling an ambulance and/or shouting). This is because in children the primary cause of the arrest is likely to be respiratory (due to a breathing problem), which may well respond favourably to a short period of BLS. In small children and infants, it may be possible to carry the child and continue BLS while you get to a telephone.

'A' IS FOR 'AIRWAY'

The airway may be blocked, and fixing this problem may be all that is necessary to save a child's life. If they are unconscious, a common cause of blockage is that the muscles of the face and jaw relax, allowing the tongue to fall backwards into the throat (or pharynx). Simple airway opening manoeuvres to lift the tongue from the back of the throat may unblock the airway, allowing the child to breathe again.

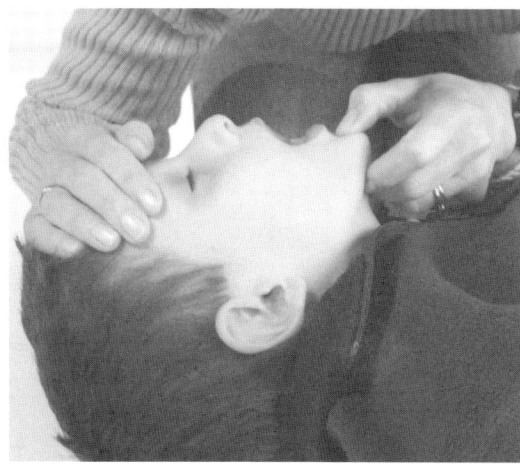

The head-tilt/chin-lift manoeuvre is used to open up the airway (see page 254).

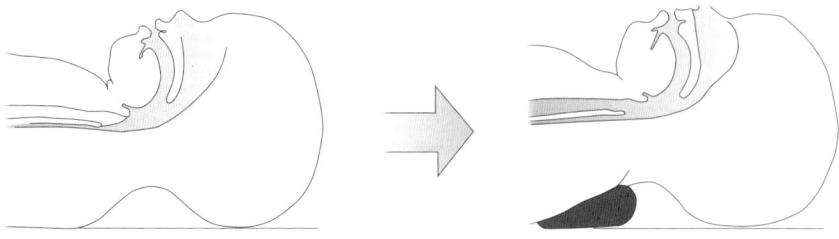

A child's larynx kinks when the head is allowed to roll forward. A towel placed under the shoulders prevents this from happening.

Opening the airway

The airway can be opened using a head-tilt/chin-lift manoeuvre. It is a two-step technique that is slightly different for infants and older children because they have differently shaped heads, and therefore the ideal head position differs with age.

1. Place one hand on the child's forehead, and apply pressure to tilt their head back gently. In infants, tilt the head to the neutral position (see diagram above). In older children, tilt the head farther back to the 'sniffing the morning air' position.
2. Place one or two fingers (depending on the size of the child) of your other hand under the bony part of the child's chin, and lift their chin upward and outward. Care should be taken not to compress or injure the soft tissues under the chin. The floor of the mouth here is very delicate and pressure from a finger may block the airway and make any obstruction worse.

Infants have large heads compared to older children and adults and this tends to push their head forward, bringing the chin onto the chest and obstructing the airway. Infants therefore need padding under their shoulders to keep the airway open (see the diagram above).

In cases where trauma (problems caused by injury rather than illness) is suspected, do not use the head-tilt/chin-lift. Instead, the jaw thrust manoeuvre (see above) should be used. This allows the neck

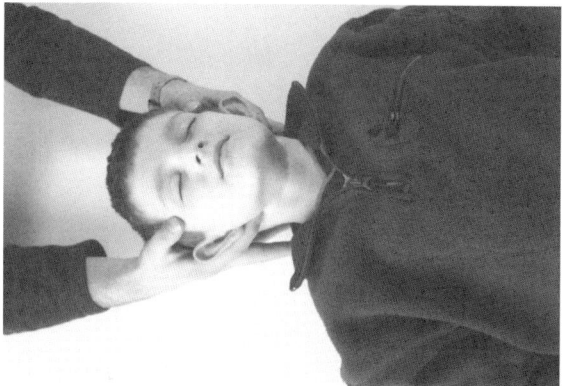

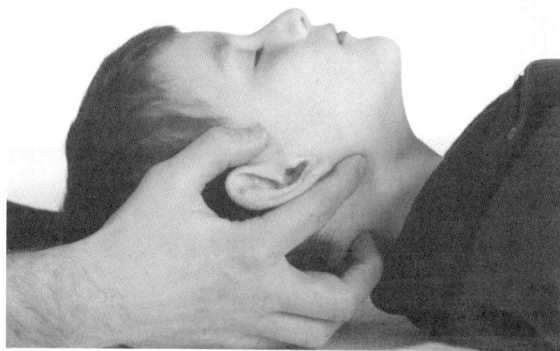

The jaw thrust manoeuvre should be used if injury is suspected. The head and neck are held in a straight line, and the airway is opened by pushing the jaw forward with the fingers.

to remain undisturbed but the airway to be opened. This is done in the following way:

- Approach the child from the top of the head. Place one hand on each side of their head, keeping the head and neck in alignment. This may be easier if your elbows are placed on the same surface as their head.
- Place two fingers of each hand under the angle of their jaw on each side. Lift the jaw upward and outward.

This jaw thrust procedure is much easier if two rescuers are present – this allows one to immobilise the child's neck and the other can open the airway.

Removing an obstruction

If any foreign material or vomit is visible in the child's mouth, then gently remove it using your finger. This should only be done if you can see the end of your finger at all times. Blind finger sweeps should not be performed because foreign material or vomit may be pushed further down the airway, causing further obstruction, and because the soft palate in children is easily damaged.

Signs the airway is open

To determine whether the airway is open, you'll need to work out whether or not the child is breathing. This is done by looking for the rise and fall of the chest, listening for breath sounds, and feeling exhaled breath against your cheek.

These three things can all be done in one position. Move your face so that your ear is over the child's nose, placing your cheek over their mouth. Look down at their chest for signs of movement, listen for breathing sounds, and try and discern the feel of their breath on your cheek. If there is no evidence of breathing after ten seconds, then you'll need to support the child's breathing.

Look — at the rise and fall of the chest. Listen — for the sound of breathing. And feel — exhaled breath against your cheek.

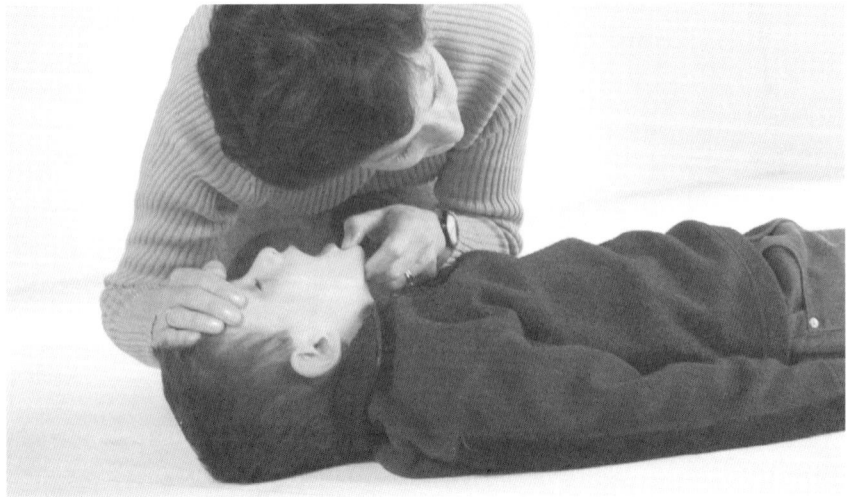

'B' IS FOR 'BREATHING'

If a child is not breathing they are not getting any oxygen into their body. Oxygen in the expired air of another person can be sufficient to keep a child alive. This is why mouth-to-mouth resuscitation is successful.

- Ensure the child's airway is open at all times using the simple airway manoeuvres outlined above.
- Breathe in and place your mouth over the child's mouth (or mouth and nose for an infant or small child), sealing it. If only the mouth is covered, their nose should be held closed with the finger and thumb of the hand holding the head.
- Slowly exhale for one second until their chest rises.

It is *very important* to remember that a child's lungs do not have the same volume as an adult's, so a full adult breath should not

When administering mouth-to-mouth resuscitation, the child's nose should be held closed with the thumb and finger of the hand holding the head.

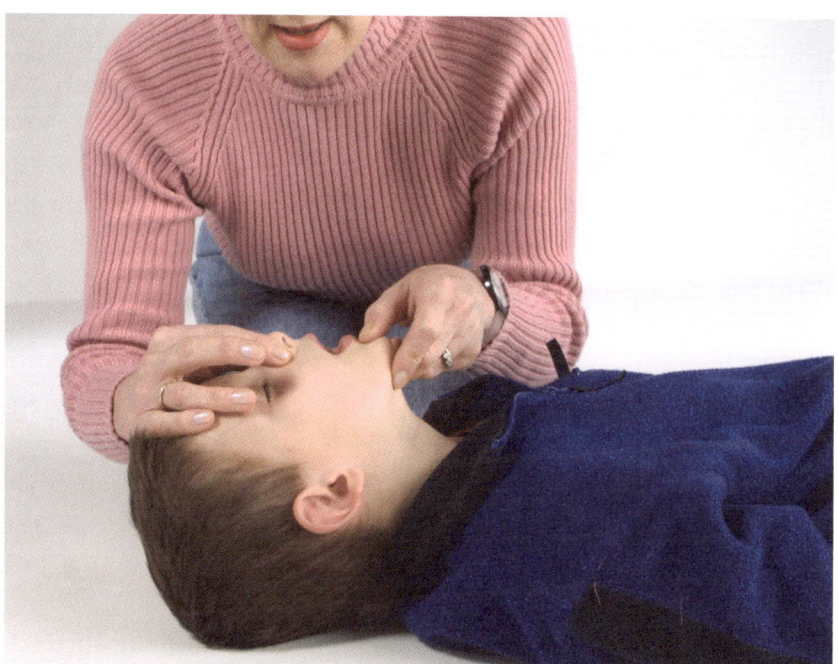

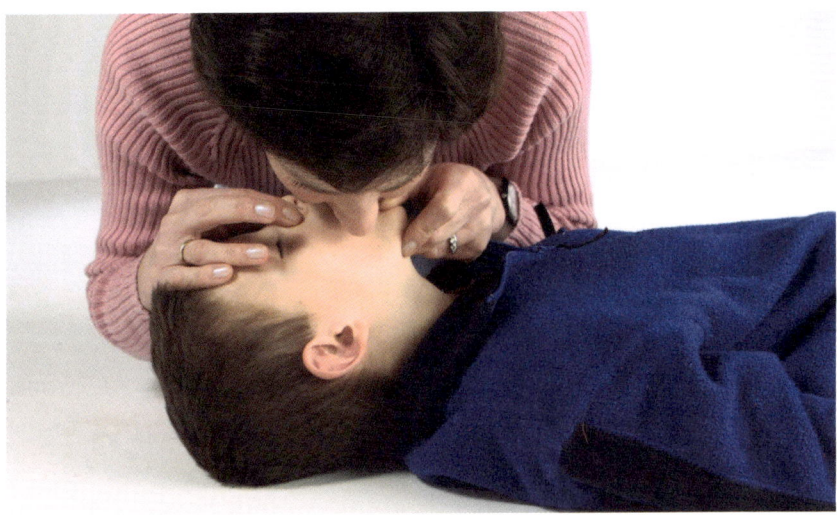

Breathe in and seal the child's mouth with your mouth, slowly exhaling until the chest rises. Initially, provide two effective breaths, with a maximum of five attempts.

be needed to inflate the child's chest. The correct volume for each breath is the amount that causes the chest to rise. Initially, provide two effective breaths, with a maximum of five attempts. This breathing must be done slowly, otherwise most of the air may go into the child's stomach rather than their lungs (and may cause them to vomit).

After the child's chest is seen to rise take a recovery breath for yourself, during which time they will passively exhale (breathe out). This recovery breath is important to keep you conscious and to increase the amount of oxygen in the next exhaled breath you give the child.

If the child's chest does not rise, then the ventilation is not effective. This could be due to the airway not being properly open, either because of poor positioning, or possibly due to a foreign body blocking the air passages. Improper opening of the airway is the commonest cause of ineffective ventilation and should be the first thing suspected if the child's chest does not rise.

The airway should be checked and opened again by reaffirming

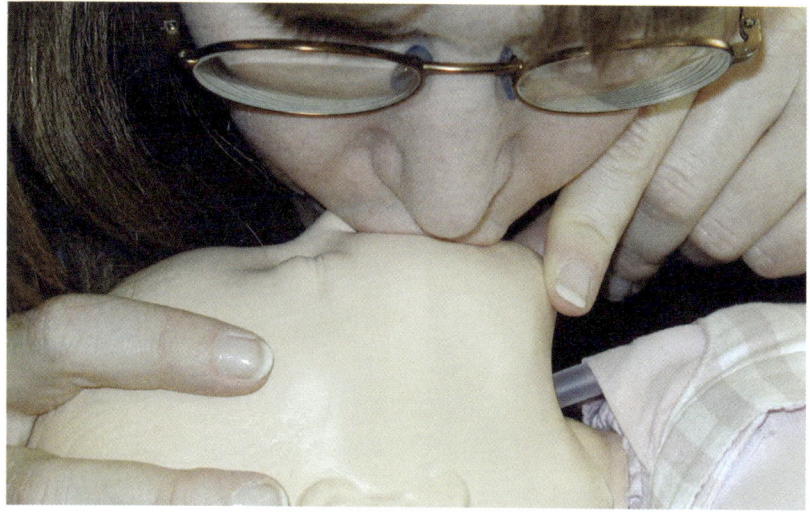

When resuscitating infants or small children, breathe into their mouth and nose, keeping the chin lifted and head tilted. Give two gentle breaths, continuing with up to five attempts, until the chest starts to rise.

the head-tilt/chin-lift position (if you are using it; see page 254). If this doesn't work, try the jaw thrust manoeuvre. If all these measures fail to clear the airway to allow effective breathing, you should suspect that a foreign body is lodged in the airway and the child is choking (see page 264).

If the child starts breathing spontaneously during these breaths, you should cease doing the mouth-to-mouth resuscitation, place them into the recovery position (see page 262) and call for help.

'C' IS FOR 'CIRCULATION'

Once the airway has been opened and two effective rescue breaths have been given, you need to assess the child's circulation. Traditionally, circulation is gauged by feeling for a pulse but studies have shown that this can be very difficult, especially in stressful circumstances, even for healthcare professionals. So if the child is moving, coughing or breathing, then their circulation is thought to be intact. But if there is no movement or obvious breathing and there is no response to any stimulation, you need to assume they are in cardiac arrest.

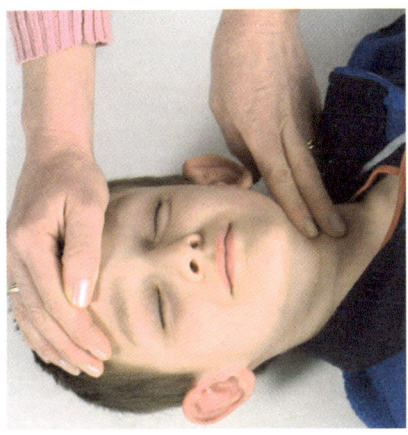 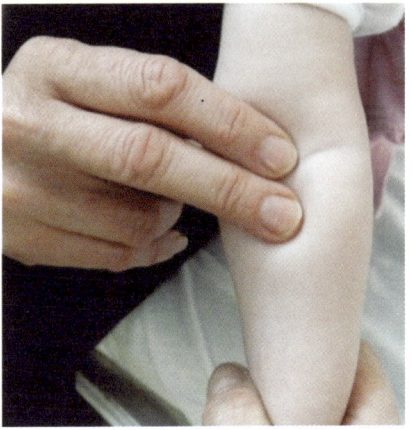

To check the pulse, feel the carotid pulse in the groove next to the Adam's apple. On an infant, feel the brachial pulse alongside the bone in the arm.

Checking the pulse

In infants, the pulse should be checked in the brachial artery, which is the large artery of the arm running alongside the inside surface of the bone. In older children, check the pulse at the carotid artery in the neck (see above). This is found by placing the fingers of one hand on the Adam's apple while maintaining head-tilt with the other, and sliding the fingers backwards into the groove made by the Adam's apple and the muscles of the neck (try it on yourself). The pulse should be easily palpable.

Check the pulse for a period of 10 seconds. If no pulse is felt, if it is slow (less than 60 beats per minute) with decreased level of consciousness or if there is absence of movement, coughing and normal breathing, then the circulation will need to be supported and chest compressions (or 'heart massage') started to maintain the pump activity of the heart and to get blood rich in oxygen around the body (see opposite).

If there is a pulse but the child is not breathing, then assisted breathing must be continued at a rate of 20 breaths per minute (or one breath every three seconds). Keep this up until either the child starts breathing again or one minute elapses. If one minute elapses and the child is still not breathing, you need to immediately call for an ambulance – 000 in Australia, 111 in New Zealand.

It is preferable that basic life support continue while you get to the telephone and call the emergency number, but if this is not possible the child must be left because help has to be summoned. Most people have mobile phones now so this can often be done simultaneously. Once you've called for help, go back to the child again and continue rescue breathing at a rate of 20 breaths per minute.

Chest compressions

People are often concerned that they may cause harm by performing CPR, but the incidence of complications as a result of resuscitation is very small in children, about 3 per cent. The results of cardiac arrest, however, are so disastrous it is always preferable to start chest compressions if there is any doubt.

To perform chest compressions, the child should be placed on a hard surface or, in the case of a small infant, they may be cradled in the crook of your forearm.

For infants and children of all ages the position for chest compressions is the lower half of the sternum (breastbone). In general, compressions should be to about a third of the depth of the child's chest. The exact technique for compressions depends on the size of the child. For an infant two fingers are used to compress the chest over the sternum. Alternatively, the infant may be held in the rescuer's hands with compressions performed using both thumbs (this is known as the hand encircling technique).

The compressions should be smooth and rhythmical, and at the end of each the pressure should be released without the fingers or hand losing contact with the chest. This prevents the need to relocate the correct position after each compression. The time taken for compression and relaxation should be approximately equal.

Once you have identified the appropriate technique, give 30 compressions and then continue assisted breathing at a ratio of two breaths then 30 compressions, repeated continuously until help arrives. You should aim for a rate of approximately 100 compressions per minute.

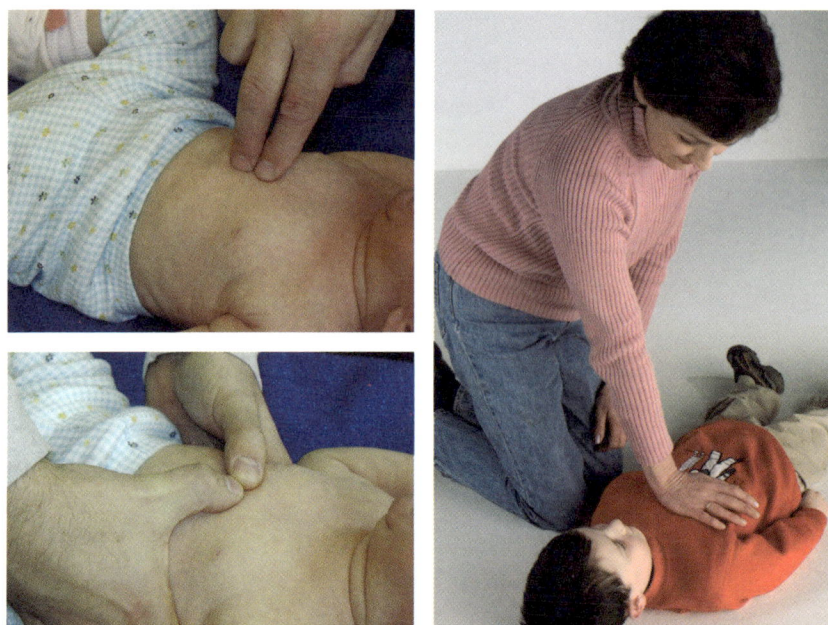

Chest compressions are performed on the lower half of the sternum, using two fingers for infants (left top) and with one hand for children (right). The hand encircling technique, using two thumbs (left bottom), may also be used for infants.

This ratio of breaths to compressions should be continued for one minute (unless the child starts breathing spontaneously). If there is still no sign of life, your next priority must be to get help by calling for an ambulance.

Once you have called the ambulance, basic life support must be resumed as soon as possible.

THE RECOVERY POSITION

If at any stage the child is breathing effectively and there is no evidence of trauma, you should place them in the recovery position, with the child lying on their side stabilised by their leg farthest from the ground (see photograph on page 263). This naturally keep the child's airway open due to gravity pulling the tongue and soft tissues of the mouth forwards, away from the back of their throat. Also, it also allows any vomit to drain away without endangering the airway.

To turn a child into the recovery position:

- kneel on their left-hand side
- tuck their left arm down the right side of their body
- cross their right arm over their chest so the right hand is hanging loosely over their left side
- use your left hand to bend the left knee up, and pull it towards you while supporting the child's head with your right hand – their head, shoulders and torso should be rolled simultaneously.

This will rotate the hips, and the body will follow with the minimum of effort. The head and neck position should be adjusted to ensure the airway is clear. To stabilise the body, bend the right knee to 90 degrees and place the right arm at 90 degrees in front of their face. Make sure the left arm is not trapped by pulling it out behind the child's torso.

The recovery position should not be used if there is any evidence of trauma, or if basic life support is still required.

To turn a child into the recovery position, kneel at the child's left hand side. Tuck the left arm down the left side of the body and the right arm over the chest and bend the right knee up.

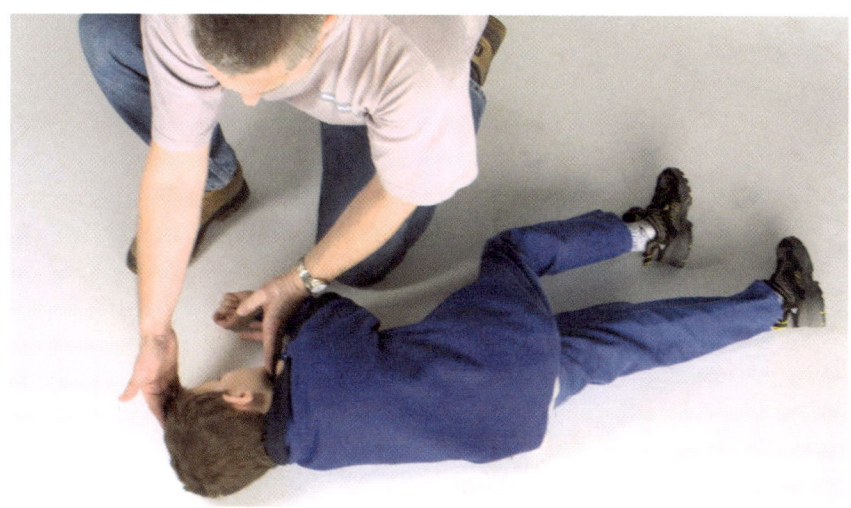

THE CHOKING CHILD

The majority of deaths of children inhaling foreign bodies occur in the pre-schoolage group. Since measures were introduced to control the minimum size of toys and toy parts for young children the incidence of this problem has decreased.

But children continue to put into their mouths almost anything they can get their hands on that fits. Predictable and potentially lethal objects, such as small toy parts, nuts and grapes, should be kept out of the reach of children.

If a child suddenly and without warning becomes very distressed, experiences breathing difficulties and starts coughing or gagging, then you should suspect they are choking. However, the symptoms of choking can be mimicked by some infections (although in infections the time taken for breathing symptoms to develop is longer.)

If you have any doubts about an apparent choking – particularly if the child had a runny nose, cough, fever, lethargy or limpness a few hours beforehand – and your child is still breathing, take them immediately to the nearest emergency department.

Attempts to dislodge a foreign body when the child has an inflamed and infected airway can make matters worse and therefore should be avoided.

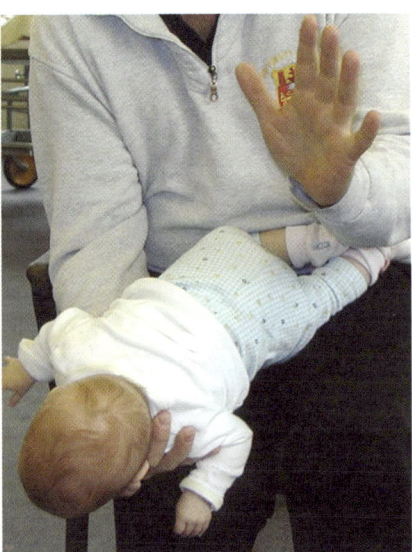

Treat a choking baby by placing the infant over your knee and giving sharp back blows between the shoulder blades.

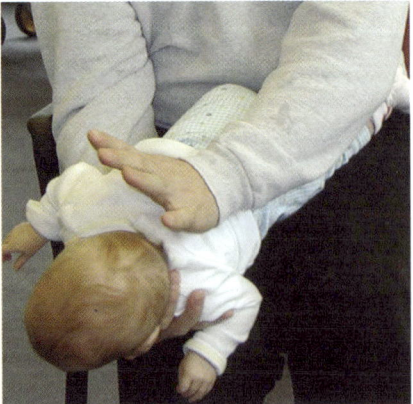

Helping the choking child

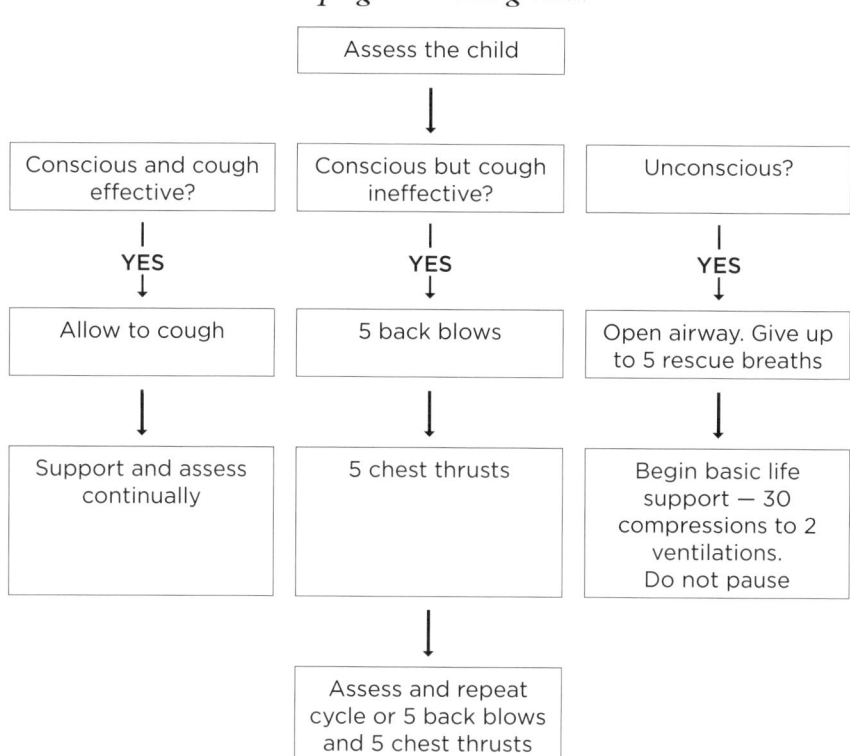

TREATMENT

The best treatment for a conscious choking child is to encourage them to expel the foreign body by coughing. For a conscious child unable to cough, it is appropriate to attempt to dislodge it for them. This is done with a combination of chest thrusts and back blows.

Back blows are given by placing the child over your knee with his head hanging down. You then hit the child in the back between the shoulder blades five times. The blow should be enough to make them fall over if they were standing – that is, it should be done quite forcefully.

If this fails, turn the child over and give them up to five sharp chest thrusts, pressing on the breastbone to a depth of about a third of the chest. Stop when the foreign body is expelled.

These chest thrusts are similar to the chest compressions described earlier, but they are sharper and are performed at a slower rate. Lay the child on their back, kneel astride them or at their feet and place the heel of one of your hands on the lower half of the sternum and then compress five times. Recheck their mouth and remove any obvious obstruction. If the first five back blows and chest thrusts are unsuccessful, then repeat the cycle of five back blows and five chest thrusts.

If the child is unconscious or stops breathing at any time, the airway should be opened and five breaths should be given using mouth-to-mouth resuscitation. Cardiopulmonary resuscitation should then be started, as described on page 261.

Once the obstruction has been relieved, the child should be placed in the recovery position and watched until help arrives.

25

HANDING OVER TO THE PROFESSIONALS

One of the most valuable things that doctors and other health professionals – paramedics who may arrive by ambulance or the triage nurse in an emergency department, for example – need when they see a patient for the first time is accurate, clear and relevant information. This information helps them to care effectively for a sick child. The 'chain of survival' starts with the first person to provide care to the child and ends with hospital care. Any interruption to this chain, even in the form of poor information, could adversely affect the child's treatment.

In general, as much information as possible should be given concerning the events leading to the emergency services being called or medical assistance sought. The majority of decisions made by doctors are formulated on the basis of this history – the story they are told concerning the event. They have the best chance of making the right decision, therefore, if they are armed with as much information as is available.

The following questions will help you put together the history of your child's illness or injury.

INFORMATION ABOUT THE ILLNESS

General information about the illness includes the following:

- What exactly is the main problem?
- When did it start?
- Was it sudden or gradual?
- When was the child last well?
- What makes the problem worse?
- What makes the problem better?
- Are there any other things that are happening as well as the main problem?
- Has anything like this happened before?
- Is the child normally well?
- Is the child completely immunised and, if not, which shots haven't they had?
- Are they on any medication (always take the medicines with you)?
- Have they ever been admitted to hospital with this or a similar problem?
- Are the rest of the family members well?

In addition to these details it is also useful to have the name and phone number of any doctor who has previously treated the child or any letter or discharge summary from a doctor or hospital.

INFORMATION ABOUT PAIN

If the problem is pain, the above questions are all important, although they are adapted specifically to the pain. Pain histories are best taken from the child herself, rather than a parent, because there may be differences you are not aware of. These are important pain questions:

- Where exactly is the pain?
- When did it start?

- Was it sudden or gradual?
- Is it constant or does it go up and down in waves (colic)?
- Is it getting worse, getting better, or staying the same?
- When did the child last feel well?
- What makes the pain worse?
- What makes the pain better?
- Does the pain go anywhere else?
- Are there any other things that are happening as well as the main problem?
- Have any painkillers been given?

INFORMATION ABOUT AN INJURY

In general, for injuries and trauma you will be expected to provide the medical personnel at the hospital with the following information about the incident:

- What are the full details of the incident?
- Was the episode witnessed and are witnesses available?
- What time did the incident occur?
- What interventions have you performed?
- What was the condition of the child when you arrived at the scene of the incident?
- Have there been any change in their condition since your arrival?

If the incident involved a motor vehicle accident, the following are vital pieces of information:

- Was the injured child a pedestrian, cyclist or passenger in a vehicle?
- If a cyclist, were they wearing a helmet?
- If a passenger, were they wearing a seatbelt or any other seat restraint?
- What speed was the car going?
- What exactly happened to the car?
- Was the child trapped in the vehicle or able to get out unaided?

- Were they ejected from the vehicle?
- Was there anyone else injured (or killed) in the accident?

INFORMATION ON RESPIRATORY OR CARDIAC ARREST

If the child has suffered a respiratory or cardiac arrest, the following information should be given:

- Was the episode witnessed?
- How long before basic life support was initiated?
- Is there any past history of medical problems?
- Recent medical problems (for example, infections, rashes, diarrhoea or vomiting, complaints of pain, any history of trauma)?
- Any change in condition since basic life support was started?

Appendices

Appendix I

YOUR HOME MEDICINE CABINET

The following is a list of items it is recommended you keep at home in your household medicine cabinet. Having a well-stocked first-aid kit is an important part of looking after the health needs of your children. But, remember, it is vitally important that your medicine cabinet is out of the reach of children and is always kept locked (make sure the key is kept in a safe but accessible place).

It is also a good idea to keep the phone number of your local poisons information centre handy – you could save it on your mobile phone or have it written on the inside door of your medicine cabinet – along with that of your GP.

INFORMATION ABOUT POISONS
Poisons Information Centre Australia: 13 11 26
Poisons Information Centre New Zealand: 0800 764 766

YOUR MEDICINE CABINET

Drugs/medicines

- Painkillers and antipyretics (to reduce fever): paracetamol (Panadol®) and ibuprofen (Nurofen®).
- Antihistamines: loratidine (Clarityn® – tablet form only), cetirizine (Zyrtec® – available as tablets or syrup).

Antihistamines should only be given for *local* allergic reactions – that is, in one area only – such as after a mosquito bite.

If you think your child has any possibility of a serious allergic reaction – swollen lips or tongue, difficulty breathing, vomiting or diarrhoea or a widespread red, itchy rash – you should seek advice from your GP or take your child to the nearest emergency department or call the emergency number (000 in Australia, 111 in New Zealand). Even if your child has a plan developed by an immunologist, part of which is antihistamine treatment, be aware that you should still use adrenaline if they have a rash and other symptoms such as shortness of breath.

Always read the dosage instructions carefully on any medicines before you give them to your children. Doses depend either on age or weight in kilograms. Ensure you know your child's correct weight. If possible, double-check the dosage with another adult or with a calculator.

Creams/lotions

- Antiseptic cream for grazes and cuts: many different brands are available but Bactroban® is the only antibiotic cream shown to be effective for most infected cuts and grazes (simply washing new cuts is usually effective).
- Calamine lotion for itchy rashes.
- Mild steroid cream for rashes – for example, Hydrazole®, which also has some antifungal action.
- Eyewash liquid to wash dirt or eyelashes out of the eyes.
- High-factor sunscreen (at least SPF 30).
- Child insect (mosquito) repellent.

Dressings and bandages

- Band-Aid® or other sticky plasters (a selection of sizes): a good fitting plaster will protect a cut or graze from becoming infected and will speed up healing.
- Crepe bandages.
- Gauze swabs.
- Medical tape – for example, Leucoplast® or Micropore®.
- Liquid Skin® – used for small cuts and grazes only.

Miscellaneous items

- Medical spoon and syringe for giving medicines – these are far more accurate than a normal teaspoon.
- Tweezers – for example, for removing splinters.
- Sterile needle – for example, for removing splinters.
- Scissors.
- Ice packs for sprains and strains.

Ice packs are best kept in the freezer, not the medicine cabinet, so that they are frozen when you need them. In place of ice packs, frozen food can be used. Anything this cold should not be applied directly to the skin because it can cause skin burns and may lower the child's body temperature too much. Wrap the ice pack in a cloth first – for example, in a tea towel.

Appendix II

GLOSSARY OF MEDICAL TERMS

Abdomen The area of the body below the chest and above the pelvis containing the stomach, bowels, liver, kidneys and other organs.

Abscess A collection of pus in an area, surrounded by inflammation. Characterised by pain, tenderness, redness, swelling.

Absence seizures A common form of childhood epilepsy, consisting of brief loss of awareness with some minimal muscle involvement. Should be distinguished from grand mal seizure.

Accessory muscles of breathing Muscles of the neck, shoulders and chest used to help the ribcage move to draw in breath in respiratory distress. Not normally needed in quiet non-distressed breathing.

Acute Of sudden onset.

Adam's apple The pointed area of the laryngeal cartilage which protects the vocal cords and which is seen in the midline at the front of the throat, especially in men.

Adrenaline A hormone produced by the adrenal glands, which lie at the top of the kidneys. Used by the body to prepare for fight or flight.

Aerobic metabolism The bodily process of breaking down foods such as sugars in the presence of oxygen. Normal way the body creates energy.

Airway The part of the respiratory anatomy through which air passes on the way to the lungs. Thought of as being from the mouth to the alveoli.

Airway opening manoeuvre Moves the jaw forward relative to the rest of the face. This pulls the tongue and floor of the mouth forward, and stops them blocking the airway in unconscious patients.

Allergy Abnormally high sensitivity to some substances, such as pollens, foods or microorganisms such as bacteria or fungi. *See* Anaphylaxis.

Altered level of consciousness Impaired awareness of surroundings, often as a result of acute illness or injury.

Alveoli Small air-containing sacs in the lungs, at the end of bronchioles. The place where oxygen from breathed-in air diffuses into the blood, and waste products such as carbon dioxide diffuse out.

Anaerobic metabolism Process of breaking down foods such as sugars in the absence of oxygen. The way the body creates energy when it cannot obtain the oxygen it needs. Produces less energy as it is much less efficient than aerobic metabolism, and creates more waste products that the body finds difficult to deal with.

Anaphylaxis A severe allergic reaction that occurs rapidly and causes a life-threatening reaction involving the whole body. *See* Allergy.

Antibiotics Medications used to treat infections due to bacteria. An example is penicillin, one of the first antibiotics. Antibiotics are probably overused as they are given for all sorts of infections; they are useless against viruses, which cause most children's infections.

Anti-inflammatory Medications that specifically target the process of inflammation, and attempt to reduce symptoms of pain, swelling, redness and local heat. Often used as effective painkillers (for example, ibuprofen).

Appendicitis Acute inflammation of the appendix, a common surgical cause of abdominal pain.

Appendix A small, worm-shaped piece of bowel in the bottom right corner of the abdomen. Has no known function. Can get inflamed, cause abdominal pain, and get taken out by surgeons.

Arterial Pertaining to an artery.

Artery A blood vessel that transports blood away from the heart, and around the body to supply oxygen to the various organs. They have muscular walls to help move the blood and contain blood at high pressures.

Aspirin Medication often used in adults as a painkiller to control temperature and to help prevent heart attacks and strokes. Should *not* be used in children as it has been implicated in development of Reye's syndrome.

Asthma A condition that causes inflammation and narrowing of the smaller airways, resulting in cough, wheeze and shortness of breath.

Back blows Firm blows to the back with the palm of hand, between the shoulder blades, in an attempt to dislodge a foreign body.

Bacterium, bacteria Type of microscopic organism, often implicated in the cause of some diseases. Responds to treatment with antibiotics.

Basic life support Treatment of suspected cardiorespiratory arrest using techniques to assess and treat problems with airway, breathing and circulation. May involve mouth-to-mouth resuscitation and CPR.

BCG Bacille Calmette-Guerin. A weakened strain of the tuberculosis bacterium, used in the vaccination against TB.

Betablockers Medication often used by adults with high blood pressure or chest pain.

Blood pressure Pressure within the arteries, made up of systolic and diastolic pressures, represented as 120/80. *See* Diastolic pressure, Systolic pressure.

Blood sugar levels Normal level of glucose carried in the blood. Glucose is used by the body as its main energy supply and is extracted from foods.

BLS *See* Basic life support.

Bone marrow Contained in central core of longer bones of the body, such as the femur, and takes part in the production of blood cells.

Bowel The part of the gastrointestinal tract between the stomach and anus. Also known as the intestine. Used by the body to extract nutrients and fluids as food passes from one end to the other.

Bronchi Either of two main branches of the trachea, leading directly to the lungs.

Bronchioles Fine, thin-walled tubular extensions of the bronchi. These lead to the alveoli.

Bronchiolitis Inflammation of the bronchioles, usually due to a virus.

Burns Injury to the skin, usually caused by heat, but also occurring after contact with some chemicals. Categorised into first, second and third degrees in terms of depth of injury.

Campylobacter Type of water-borne bacterium that is frequently implicated in the development of diarrhoea.

Capillaries The smallest vessels containing oxygenated blood. They allow red blood cells to travel in single file and are responsible for delivering oxygen to the tissues on a cellular level.

Carbohydrates A prime source of nutrition for the body. This type of food includes sugars and starches.

Carbon dioxide A gas, a waste product of respiration, transported from the body's cells by the blood and breathed out in the lungs.

Carbon monoxide A colourless, odourless, highly poisonous gas often produced from the incomplete combustion of substances. It prevents oxygen from combining with haemoglobin.

Cardiac arrest The complete cessation of spontaneous heartbeat. In children usually result of prolonged period of respiratory illness or fluid loss. Also known as cardiopulmonary or cardiorespiratory arrest.

Cardiac massage Process of using hands to repeatedly press on the chest of a person with cardiac arrest, in order to provide pumping action to move blood around the body.

Cardiopulmonary resuscitation Process of attempting to maintain function of the airway, breathing and circulation in a patient with cardiac arrest. Involves mouth-to-mouth resuscitation and cardiac massage, to provide partially oxygenated air to the lungs and some heart pumping action to move blood round the body.

Cardiovascular system Consists of heart, arteries, capillaries and veins, which together move blood carrying oxygen and nutrients to the body tissues, and carbon dioxide and other waste products away from them.

Carotid artery The large artery that supplies blood to the head.

Cartilage A tough, elastic connective tissue found largely in joints.

Cells The smallest structural unit of an organism that is capable of independent functioning.

Cervical spine Area of the spine connecting the head to the chest. This area is particularly vulnerable in trauma because of its flexibility.

Chest compressions *See* Cardiac massage.

Chest thrusts Method of removing a foreign body by pressing quickly on the chest in attempt to push it out by suddenly increasing the pressure in the lungs and airway. Similar movement to cardiac massage.

Chicken pox Acute contagious disease, primarily of children, caused by the varicella–zoster virus and characterised by skin eruptions, slight fever and malaise.

Cholera Acute infectious disease of the small intestine, caused by a bacterium and characterised by profuse watery diarrhoea, vomiting, muscle cramps and severe dehydration.

Chromosomal abnormality Abnormality that produces defective chromosomes, often as a result of problems in the combination of different strands of DNA, which occurs during fertilisation of an egg by a sperm.

Chromosomes (*aka* Genes). Parts of a strand of specialised protein known as DNA, which carries all the information necessary for cells to reproduce and form the organs of the body.

Circulation Movement of blood through vessels as a result of the heart's pumping action.

Circulatory failure Failure of the cardiovascular system to supply adequate amounts of blood to body tissues. May be due to loss of the heart's pumping action, insufficient amounts of blood or failure of the blood vessels to maintain pressure in the system.

Clinical sign Objective evidence of disease visible to examining doctor.

Cold sore Scabbed area on the lips, with groups of watery blisters on the skin, caused by infection of the herpes simplex virus, which lies dormant in nerves leading to the area.

Coma A deep prolonged unconsciousness from which the patient cannot be roused.

Common cold Viral upper respiratory tract infection. Contagious illness. Because of the great number of different types of viruses that can cause a cold, the body never builds up immunity against all of them. For this reason, colds are a frequent and recurring problem. Preschool children average nine colds a year, those in kindergarten 12, and adolescents and adults seven. Going out in cold weather has no effect on the spread of a cold. Antibiotics do not help.

Compression bandage A dressing that stops the flow of blood from a bleeding area by applying pressure.

Congenital A condition present at birth.

Connective tissue Material forming the supporting and connecting tissues of the body

Contagious *See* Infection.

Convulsion Series of violent involuntary muscular contractions, often followed by relaxation. Also known as seizure or fit.

Cot death *See* Sudden Infant Death Syndrome.

Cough reflex Reflex that makes one cough when the airways are irritated.

CPR Cardiopulmonary resuscitation.

Cross-infection Infection transmitted between individuals infected by different microscopic organisms.

Croup Often occurs after a child contracts a viral upper respiratory tract infection. Results in inflammation and increased production of mucus. Parents often describe a barking or seal-like cough. Difficulty in breathing can be quite marked, and may result in stridor. Children often need to be assessed in an emergency department.

Cyanosis Bluish discolouration, especially of the lips and other mucous membranes. Usually a result of blood that has poor oxygen content.

Dehydration Relative lack of fluid in the body compared with the normal state. Often as a result of losing liquid in a fever, as sweat and as evaporated water in breathing, and in gastrointestinal problems, as vomit and diarrhoea. Can be dangerous, especially in small children, as the normal processes of the body start to fail if a child is too dehydrated.

Diabetes Disease that makes the body unable to process and use the sugars obtained in food. Diabetes is due to a lack of a hormone called insulin, which controls this process.

Diaphragm The sheet of very thin muscle that divides the abdominal cavity of the body (containing the stomach, intestines, kidneys etc.) from the thoracic cavity, or chest (containing the heart and lungs). It takes part in breathing by increasing the volume of the chest and lungs.

Diarrhoea Passage of excessive number of fluid faeces.

Diastolic pressure The figure on the bottom half of a blood pressure measurement – for example, the '80' in 120/80 – which represents the baseline pressure in the arteries between heartbeats.

DNA Deoxyribonucleic acid. Strands of specialised protein which carry all the information necessary for cells to reproduce and form the organs of the body.

Eardrum A thin membrane stretched across the ear passage separating the external ear canal from the middle ear. Contains the mechanisms of hearing.

Ecstasy (*aka* MDMA). Street drug combining a stimulant, which gives increased sense of energy, with a hallucinogen, which improves mood; often used for all-night dance parties. Long-term use may cause damage to brain's ability to regulate sleep, pain, memory and emotions.

Eczema Non-contagious inflammation of the skin characterised by redness, itching and outbreak of lesions which may discharge serous matter and become encrusted and scaly.

Encephalitis Inflammation of the brain.

Epiglottis Flap of tissue that folds down when swallowing to protect the airway from the entry of food and fluid.

Epilepsy Disorder of the central nervous system commonly characterised by loss of consciousness and convulsions. May exist in a form which only affects one area of the body. *See* Convulsion.

Exhale, expiration To breathe out; to expel air from the lungs.

External respiration The exchange of oxygen and carbon dioxide between the environment and the lungs.

Faeces Waste products formed in the bowel from digestion of food.

Fats Any of various soft, solid or semisolid compounds, found in animal and plants. One of the essential components of the diet.

Febrile convulsions A brief seizure associated with fever, lasting less than 15 minutes, seen in an otherwise neurologically normal infant or child.

Femur The largest bone of the leg, running from the hip to knee.

Fever A rise in body temperature above normal, often as a response to infection. Typically thought of as oral temperature above 38°C.

Finger sweeps Use of a finger to sweep around the inside of mouth and pharynx to remove any foreign bodies. The technique is *not* recommended for children when it cannot be performed under direct vision.

Fit *See* Convulsion.

Floppy baby A baby with poor muscle tone unable to maintain normal posture. Usually the mark of an extremely ill child, and requires emergency assessment by a doctor in an emergency department. Should be transported by emergency ambulance.

Foreign body Substance occurring in any part of the body where it does not belong, and usually introduced from outside.

Fractures Breaks in a bone.

Gas exchange Process of exchange of oxygen for carbon dioxide at the lungs.

Gastrointestinal tract The digestive system, stretching from the mouth to the anus. Consisting of the oesophagus, stomach, small intestine, large intestine, and all associated organs, such as the liver, spleen and pancreas.

Genetic makeup The design for an individual, contained on the chromosomes in the nucleus of the body's cells.

Glue ear Chronic (long-term) condition in which there is a secretion of thick fluid into the middle ear. Commonest cause of hearing loss in children and may interfere with normal speech development and cause learning difficulties.

Golden hour The time immediately after a trauma occurs, when the consequences of the injury can be minimised by correct and urgent treatment.

Grand mal seizure Name for a convulsion involving the whole body, associated with a loss of consciousness.

Greenstick Type of fracture that often occurs in children, when the bone bends but only fractures on one side; said to be similar to a young tree branch.

Grommet Plastic device shaped like a cotton reel placed in eardrum of children with glue ear to provide circulating air to the middle ear.

Haemoglobin Red-coloured protein carried in red blood cells, used to transport oxygen around the body. Oxygen bonds to the haemoglobin, turning the colour of the blood from dark red in the veins coming from the body to the lungs to bright red in the arteries travelling in the opposite direction.

Hay fever Inflammatory response to allergic stimulus, often pollen or other plant products. Usually results in nasal congestion and sneezing.

Head-tilt/chin-lift Manoeuvre used to open the airway of a child in basic life support, when there is no evidence of any trauma.

Hepatitis B Severe viral infection of the liver, transmitted in blood and other bodily fluids. Very infectious and may be carried in the body without symptoms. A vaccine is available.

Herpes simplex *See* Cold sore.

HIV Human Immunodeficiency Virus. The infective organism that causes AIDS.

Hives (*aka* Urticaria) Allergic skin rash characterised by multiple smooth, raised pink areas that can develop suddenly anywhere on the body.

Hoarseness An unnaturally deep or rough quality of the voice.

Hole-in-the-heart Term for congenital heart problem: defect in the muscle wall between two chambers of the heart. May be associated with other defects, such as incorrect positioning of blood vessels running to and from heart. May be corrected by surgery early in life.

Hypothermia Subnormal temperature of the body. Usually taken as temperature below 35°C. If not corrected may cause major problems with cardiovascular and other systems. Children are more prone to it than adults as they have a large body surface area and relatively small volume, thus can lose heat easily. Young babies are unable to compensate for cold by shivering, thus even more prone to hypothermia.

Ibuprofen Anti-inflammatory medication usually used as a painkiller or to decrease temperature in a fever. Available at chemists without prescription. Commonly seen under the brand name Nurofen©.

Immobilisation Practice of maintaining the neck in stable, stationary position after a trauma to minimise possible cervical spine injury.

Immune system Body's defences against infection, comprising a variety of cells that fight off invading microorganisms.

Immunisation programs Programs designed to eradicate serious infectious diseases from a community. Consist of single or multiple vaccines against a particular infecting organism, usually given early in life. Vaccines are usually made of organisms that have been killed, and thus cannot cause infection but can stimulate the immune response, or inactivated segments of the poisons, that the organisms produce.

Immunity Ability to resist diseases caused by infective microorganisms. Passed on from mother to baby, acquired through exposure to organisms throughout life, or conferred by immunisation programs.

Infant A child under the age of one year.

Infection Invasion by, and multiplication of, pathogenic microorganisms in part of the body or tissue. May produce subsequent tissue injury and progress to overt disease through a variety of cellular or toxic mechanisms.

Inflammation A localised protective reaction of tissue to irritation, injury or infection characterised by pain, redness, swelling and sometimes loss of function.

Influenza Acute contagious viral infection characterised by inflammation of respiratory tract and by fever, chills, and muscular pain.

Inhale To breathe in, to draw air into the lungs.

Inhaler Device containing medication in a pressurised liquid form, which is released in a metered amount as a spray when the activating button is depressed. Commonly used to treat asthma in children.

Inspiration *See* Inhale.

Insulin Natural hormone produced by the pancreas that aids in the metabolism and storage of sugars and fats. Given as an injected medication in some forms of diabetes when it is not produced naturally.

Intercostal muscles Muscles between the ribs that take part in breathing by expanding the chest.

Internal respiration Process of metabolism of foods in the cells, either with or without oxygen.

Iron supplement Medication to help increase amount of haemoglobin produced to ensure sufficient transport of oxygen from the lungs to the tissues.

Irritable bowel syndrome A disorder characterised by abnormally increased movement of the small and large intestinal contents, producing abdominal pain, constipation or diarrhoea.

Jaw thrust Manoeuvre used in basic life support to open the airway when there is a suspicion of neck trauma.

Large airways The trachea and bronchi.

Larynx The part of the airway partway down the trachea, which protects and supports the vocal cords.

Level of consciousness Level of awareness of the surroundings. Ranges from conscious (fully aware and awake) to unconscious.

Ligament A band of fibrous tissue connecting bones and cartilages serving to reinforce and strengthen joints.

Liver A large organ in the upper right of the abdomen with multiple functions. Involved in the storage of food, production of proteins, clotting of blood and detoxification of harmful substances.

Lower respiratory tract Bronchi, bronchioles and lungs.

Lower respiratory tract infection (LRTI) Infection, often caused by a virus, of the lower respiratory tract.

Lymphoid tissue Areas involved in the production and storage of various types of white blood cells.

Malaise A vague feeling of bodily discomfort, as at the start of an illness.

Mastoiditis Inflammation of the mastoid process, the bony area behind the ear that contains cavities filled with air.

Measles Acute, contagious viral disease usually occurring in childhood. Characterised by eruption of red spots on the skin, fever and inflammation of mucous membranes, especially of nose and throat.

Membrane A thin, pliable layer of tissue covering surfaces or separating or connecting regions, structures or organs. Also refers to the outer layer of cells.

Meninges The three layers of membrane lining the inside of the skull and outside of the brain. Sometimes infected by microorganisms to cause the condition known as meningitis.

Meningitis Inflammation of the meninges of the brain and spinal cord, most often caused by bacterial or viral infection and characterised by fever, vomiting, intense headache and stiff neck. In children some of these symptoms, especially headache and stiff neck, might be absent.

Metabolic rate Rate at which energy is produced from food.

Metabolism Process of producing energy by the body from ingested food.

Middle ear The bony chamber containing the mechanisms of hearing, separated from the external ear canal by the eardrum.

Migraine A severe recurring headache, usually affecting only one side of the head, characterised by sharp pain and often accompanied by nausea, vomiting and visual disturbances.

MMR vaccine Measles, mumps and rubella vaccine. Contains three separate vaccines in one injection; protects against measles, mumps and rubella (German measles). Is given at 13 or 15 months of age and again before children go to school. The second dose protects those who did not respond to the first dose. A link between the measles vaccine and inflammatory bowel disease or autism has been suggested. Research on this issue has been reviewed by experts from around the world, including the World Health Organization, and on all the evidence available they have agreed that there is no link between MMR and autism.

Mouth-to-mouth Method of artificial ventilation involving covering the patient's mouth (and nose in small children) with the rescuer's mouth to inflate the patient's lungs by blowing. This is followed by a period of unassisted expiration caused by recoil of the patient's chest.

Mucous membrane Moist lubricated inner lining of the mouth, nose, gut and urethra. This membrane lines the inner surface of all organs containing mucus-secreting glands.

Mumps Infectious acute viral disease affecting the parotid salivary glands, gonads, meninges and pancreas. Common symptoms may include weakness, fever, sore throat, malaise and puffy cheeks due to the parotid gland swelling. Patients are contagious one day prior to the onset of swelling and continue to be contagious until the swelling is gone, usually in approximately two weeks.

Nasal flaring Widening of the nostrils with inspiration, in a child having difficulty in breathing. A marker of respiratory distress.

Nebuliser Method of delivering liquid medication by bubbling high-flow oxygen through it via a specially designed chamber attached to an oxygen mask. Used for treating asthma. Children are often treated by multiple puffs of an inhaler via a spacer instead.

Neurological Relating to the brain or nervous system.

Occiput The back part of the head or skull.

Oesophagus (*aka* the gullet) Muscular membranous tube for the passage of food from the pharynx to stomach.

Oral rehydration solutions Fluids that contain correct proportions of essential chemicals and nutrients to replace the body fluids lost in dehydration, diarrhoea and vomiting.

Oxygen A clear gas that is essential for life. Used in the metabolism of foods in the cells to give the body energy. Complete lack of oxygen for a relatively short time will result in death.

Pacemaker An area of specialised heart muscle that is able to initiate a heartbeat and has its own intrinsic rhythm. Various areas of the heart are able to do this in an emergency, but much less efficiently and at a much slower rate than the pacemaker cells.

Paracetamol Common medication often used for the relief of minor to moderate pain, and to decrease body temperature in infectious conditions leading to fever. Commonly found in children's preparations such as Calpol. Very dangerous in overdose so keep to maximum dose recommended on the packaging or by a doctor.

Penicillin One of the first antibiotics discovered, still in common use.

Pertussis *See* Whooping cough.

Pharynx The section of digestive tract extending from the mouth and nasal cavities to the larynx, where it becomes continuous with the oesophagus.

Phlegm Thick, sticky, stringy mucus secreted by mucous membrane of respiratory tract, as during a cold or other respiratory infection.

Pleurisy Inflammation of the linings around the lungs, or pleura, usually occurring as a complication of a disease such as pneumonia, accompanied by an accumulation of fluid in the pleural cavity, chills, fever, and painful breathing and coughing.

Pneumonia An acute or chronic disease marked by inflammation of the lungs and caused by viruses, bacteria or other microorganisms and sometimes by physical or chemical irritants.

Posseting An effortless return of stomach contents into the mouth. Common in children in the first year of life when a small amount of milk or feed comes back up. It results from immaturity of the ring of muscle at the lower end of the oesophagus.

Protein One of the basic types of food, used in building muscle and other tissues. Examples of foods high in protein are meat and fish.

Pulse The palpable sensation of blood passing through an artery close to the skin, occurring with every heartbeat. Most commonly felt at the wrist, upper arm (especially in babies) and neck, where the carotid artery passes to the head.

Pus Yellow-green liquid exuded from infected wounds or abscesses. By-product of infection and inflammation, composed of dead white blood cells that have attacked and killed invading organisms.

Rate of breathing Number of breaths taken in a minute. A good marker of respiratory distress. May be counted by looking at a watch, counting the breaths in 15 seconds and multiplying by four.

Recovery breath A breath taken by a rescuer performing mouth-to-mouth resuscitation, which increases the amount of oxygen in the rescuer's exhaled air and thus increases the amount delivered to the child with the next breath.

Recovery position Position in which person's airway is naturally held open due to gravity pulling the tongue and soft tissues of the mouth forward, away from the back of the throat. The patient lies on the side, stabilised by the leg farthest from the ground.

Reflux *See* Posseting.

Rescue breathing Part of basic life support, using five attempts to give two effective mouth-to-mouth breaths. The rescuer breathes in then seals their mouth over the child's mouth (or mouth and nose of an infant or small child), and slowly exhales over one or two seconds until the patient's chest is seen to rise. While doing this, if only the mouth is covered, the nose is held closed with the finger and thumb of the hand holding the head.

Respiratory distress When difficulty in breathing becomes severe. Should be assessed by looking at the effort and effectiveness of breathing: the rate of breathing, signs of nasal flaring or accessory muscle use, and whether the patient can talk in sentences, is pale, sweaty, drowsy or cyanosed.

Respiratory infection Very common cause of illness in children. May affect upper respiratory tract (URTI), including mouth, nose, pharynx, ears and tonsils, or lower respiratory tract (LRTI), including bronchi, bronchioles and lungs. Commonly caused by viruses but may be caused by bacteria in more severe cases.

Respiratory rate *See* Rate of breathing.

Rubella (*aka* German measles) Mild contagious rash-forming disease caused by a virus. Capable of producing congenital defects in infants born to mothers infected during first three months of pregnancy.

Salbutamol Medication, known as a bronchodilator, used to treat asthma. Given by inhaler or nebuliser, assists in relaxing and opening up bronchi and bronchioles. Type of medication also known as reliever.

Salmonella Type of bacteria sometimes implicated in food poisoning. Can be associated with quite severe diarrhoea and dehydration.

Scalds Burns due to hot fluids or steam.

Seizure *See* Convulsion.

Sepsis Severe infective condition, where infecting organisms spread to the blood and affect organs such as the lungs, heart and kidneys.

Shock Medical condition where there is insufficient oxygenated blood being supplied to the tissues, especially the vital organs. Usually caused by bleeding, infection or heart problems. Not to do with 'being shocked' by a frightening or upsetting event.

SIDS *See* Sudden Infant Death Syndrome.

Signs Objective evidence of a disease – that is, something seen or perceived such as swelling or a rash.

Smallpox Severe viral disease with a high mortality rate. Officially eradicated worldwide in 1979 through vaccination programs.

Smoke inhalation Common cause of death in house fires. Smoke contains carbon monoxide and other noxious substance; the colourless, odourless gas removes oxygen from haemoglobin in the blood so the body's cells and tissues do not get enough oxygen to function.

'Sniffing the morning air' The position to place an older child's head and neck in when doing the head-tilt/chin-lift manoeuvre.

Soft palate The posterior part of the roof of the mouth.

Soft tissues Skin, muscle, fat and soft connective tissues.

Spacer A cylindrical plastic chamber that fits onto an inhaler. Several puffs of medication are squirted into the chamber, and the child breathes it in. Method of giving inhaled medication that is efficient and easy for parents and children.

Spasm Sudden involuntary contraction of a muscle or a group of muscles, sometimes associated with pain.

Spleen An organ situated on the left side of the abdomen, near the stomach. Part of the immune system.

Splinting Immobilising a fractured or sprained limb, by attaching it to a rigid object, such as a stick or another limb, to reduce movement and discomfort at the fracture site.

Sprains A tearing injury to ligaments. Can be minor, with only a slight stress to the ligament, or severe with complete separation of a ligament that supports a joint.

Steroid Substance that occurs naturally in the body as a hormone and has many uses. Artificial versions are often used medically in the treatment of asthma and croup to suppress inflammation.

Stomach ulcers Ulcer occurring in membrane lining the stomach.

Strains A tearing injury to muscle. Usually results in some bleeding into the muscle tissues.

Stridor Harsh sound made on inhalation through a narrowed airway. Indicates a partial blockage. The child needs to be seen by doctor immediately.

Sudden Infant Death Syndrome (*aka* SIDS) Defined as the sudden death of an infant less than one year of age. Even after a thorough case investigation, including autopsy, examination of death scene and review of clinical history, the death remains unexplained.

Symptoms Subjective evidence of a disease – that is, something felt or perceived by the patient, such as abdominal pain or headache.

Systolic pressure The figure on the top half of a blood pressure measurement – the '120' in 120/80 – representing the peak pressure in the arteries when the heart beats.

Tachypnoea A rate of breathing faster than normal for the size and age of the child.

TB *See* Tuberculosis.

Tendon A fibrous, strong tissue that connects muscle to bone.

Tetanus An acute, often fatal, disease caused by bacterium, which often enters the body through contaminated puncture wounds such as those caused by nails, splinters and insect bites. A vaccine is available as part of the routine childhood immunisation program.

Thorax Anatomical name for the chest. Contains the heart and lungs, and is separated from the abdominal cavity by the diaphragm.

Tissue A group of similar cells united to perform a similar function – for example, the liver is made up of specialised tissue, all of which perform the same function.

Tonsillitis Inflammation of the tonsils, usually due to an infection.

Tonsils Collection of lymphoid tissue covered by mucous membrane, located on either side of the rear of the mouth at the junction with the pharynx.

Torso The human trunk.

Toxicity The potential for a substance to act as a toxin.

Toxin Poisonous substance that is a specific product of the metabolic activities of a living organism. Usually very unstable, notably toxic when introduced into the tissues, and typically capable of inducing the formation of antibodies.

Trachea The part of the airway from the epiglottis to the bronchi. The largest part of the airway.

Trauma Accidental injury.

Triage To sort. The process used in an emergency department to prioritise which patients are seen first – for example, a fitting child will be seen before a child with a minor injury.

Tricyclic anti-depressant Type of anti-depression medication. Particularly dangerous in overdose as it may cause abnormal heart rhythms and convulsions, which may be fatal.

Tripoding A child in respiratory distress who sits upright on the edge of the bed with arms outstretched, hands on knees. They are using the position of their chest wall to facilitate breathing.

Tuberculosis (*aka* TB) A disease caused by a microorganism and transmitted from person to person by tiny droplets in coughs and sneezes. Previously a major killer but rate of deaths had declined markedly due to immunisation programs and effective antibiotics. Unfortunately, it is starting to become more common again.

Ulcer A circumscribed area of eroded tissue, often due to inflammation.

Upper respiratory tract/passages Mouth, nose, pharynx, ears and tonsils.

Upper respiratory tract infection (URTI) Infection, often caused by a virus, of the upper respiratory tract, including the mouth, nose, pharynx, ears and tonsils.

Urinary tract infection (UTI) Bacterial infection of the bladder, urethra, ureters or kidneys (the urinary tract). Symptoms are pain on urination, urgency, frequency, fever and often vomiting in children. Children with a first urinary tract infection need further investigation. Should be treated with antibiotics.

Urticaria *See* Hives.

Vaccine A suspension of weakened or dead microorganisms which stimulate the immune system to produce antibodies against the specific genuine disease. *See* Immunisation programs.

Varicella–zoster virus Virus causing chicken pox.

Veins Thin-walled blood vessels that carry blood, which is low in oxygen but high in waste products, from body tissues back to the heart and lungs.

Viruses Microorganism with only a central DNA strand and a protein coat land on and infect cells, causing a number of diseases.

Vital organs The organs essential to maintain life. Includes the brain, heart, lungs, liver and kidneys.

Vomiting The sudden involuntary expulsion of stomach contents through the oesophagus and mouth.

White blood cells (WBCs) Cells that combat invading microorganisms by directly killing them and by stimulating the immune system to produce antibodies against the particular type of organism.

Whooping cough A highly contagious bacterial infection of the respiratory system, usually affecting children, caused by a bacterium. Characterised in the advanced stage by spasms of coughing interspersed with deep, noisy whooping inspirations. Increasingly rare due to an effective immunisation program. Can be mild to severe. Symptoms include a runny nose, fever, sore eyes and a cough.

X-rays Type of radiation that passes through the body and creates a negative photographic image on specially sensitised film. Good technique for looking at bones and bony injuries such as fractures. Not always needed in injury, particularly soft-tissue injuries. They are not harmful unless one is exposed to a great number of them; however, precautions are always taken to safeguard against unnecessary exposure, especially of children or pregnant women.

Useful information and addresses

BITES, STINGS AND POISONS

Australian Museum: <www.austmus.gov.au/factsheets>

Australian Resuscitation Council guideline 8.9.1. Envenomation – pressure immobilisation technique

Australian Resuscitation Council guideline 8.9.6. Envenomation – jellyfish stings

Poisons Information Centre Australia: 13 11 26

Poisons Information Centre New Zealand: 0800 764 766

BREATHING DIFFICULTIES

All Health Australia, bronchiolitis: <www.allhealth.com.au/html/s02_article/article_view.asp?keyword=bronchiolitis>

Asthma and Respiratory Foundation New Zealand:

Children's Hospital Westmead, whooping cough: <www.chw.edu.au/parents/factsheets/reswhooj.htm>

National Asthma Council Australia: <www.nationalasthma.org.au>

Parenting and Child Health, croup: <www.cyh.com/HealthTopics/HealthTopicDetails.aspx?p=114&np=304&id=18544>

HEARING

Advice on hearing testing Australian Hearing, phone 13 17 97

National Foundation for the Deaf, New Zealand: <www.nfd.org.nz>

Deaf societies in Australia and New Zealand Most states and cities have their own deaf societies that are good sources of information for parents and children with hearing problems – for example, <www.auckland-deaf.org.nz> and <www.deafsocietynsw.org.au>.

IMMUNISATION

Further information about the facts behind immunisation can be found at <www.immunise.health.gov.au> and <www.immune.org.nz>.

The Immunise Australia Program: <www.immunise.health.gov.au/internet/immunise/pushling.nsf/Contents/nips>

Australian state and territory vaccination information

ACT: (02) 6205 2300

NSW: Contact the local Public Health Units (look under 'Health' in the White Pages)

NT: (09) 8922 8315

QLD: (07) 3234 1500

SA: (08) 8226 7177

Tas: 1800 671 738 (from Tasmania only), (03) 6222 7724 (outside Tasmania)

Vic: 1300 882 008

WA: (08) 9321 1312

INFECTIONS

Parenting and Child Health, croup: <www.cyh.com/HealthTopics/HealthTopicDetails.aspx?p=114&np=304&id=18544>

Children's Hospital Westmead, whooping cough: <www.chw.edu.au/parents/factsheets/reswhooj.htm>

All Health Australia, bronchiolitis: <www.allhealth.com.au/html/s02_article/article_view.asp?keyword=bronchiolitis>

INJURY PREVENTION

Useful information on child safety and accident prevention: <www.rospa.com>

Australian Transport Safety Bureau, 'A simple guide to child restraints': <www.atsb.gov.au>

Child Safety Foundation, New Zealand: <www.childsafety.co.nz>

Children's Hospital Westmead: <www.chw.edu.au/parents/factsheets>

Kidshealth New Zealand: <www.kidshealth.org.nz>

Kidslife, 'Make your home and garden safe for children': <www.kidslife.com.au>

Kidsafe Australia: <www.kidsafe.com.au>

New Zealand Transport Agency, 'Factsheet 7: Child Restraints':
  <www.landtransport.govt.nz/factsheets/07.html>
Safe Kids New Zealand: <www.safekids.org.nz>
Safe Kids Worldwide: <www.safekids.org>
Sydney Children's Hospital: <www.sch.edu.au/health/factsheets/>
Royal Children's Hospital, Melbourne, 'Safety and your child':
  <www.rch.org.au/kidsinfo/factsheets.ctm>

MENTAL HEALTH
ADHD
ADHD Australia: <www.adhd.com.au>
ADHD.org New Zealand: <www.adhd.org.nz/>

Autism
Autismhelpinfo: <www.autismhelp.info/main.htm>,
Spectrum Australia: <www.aspect.org.au>

Eating disorders
Anorexia Bulimia Help: <www.anorexiabulimiahelp.com/>
Australia Health: <www.australiahealth.com/Healthinformation/
  HealthConditions/anorexia.htm>
Eating Disorders Association of New Zealand: <www.ed.org.nz/
  index.asp?pageID=2145862939>
NSW Health advice: <www.health.nsw.gov.au/topics/anorexia.
  html>
Victorian Government Health Information: <www.health.vic.gov.
  au/mentalhealth/illnesses/eating>

Drug use
Parents. The Anti drug: <www.theantidrug.com/>
About.com: Teens: <parentingteens.about.com/od/teendruguse>
MedicineNet.com: <www.medicinenet.com/teen_drug_abuse/
  article.htm>

Notes

INTRODUCTION
R Crampton, 'The problem of cardiac arrest in the community', *Amer J Emergency Med*, 2(3): 204–9, May 1984.

CHAPTER 5: INFECTIONS
ABC of One to Seven, BMJ Books, 2000.
American Academy of Paediatrics guidelines: <www.aap.org/ advocacy/releases/aomqa.htm>.

CHAPTER 6: FEVERS
E Autret-Leca, et al., 'Ibuprofen versus paracetamol in paediatric fever: objective and subjective findings from a randomised, blinded study', *Curr Med Res Opin*, 23(9): 2205, September 2007.
MD Erlewyn-Lajeunesse, et al., 'Randomised controlled trial of combined paracetamol and ibuprofen for fever', *Arch Dis Child*, 91: 414, May 2006.
Royal Children's Hospital Melbourne, 'Fever in children': <www.rch. org.au/kidsinfo/factsheets.cfm?doc_id=5200>.
AD Wright, et al., 'Alternating antipyretics for fever reduction in children: and unfounded practice passed down to parents from paediatricians', *Clin Ped*, 46(2): 146, March 2007.

CHAPTER 7: BREATHING DIFFICULITES
The British Thoracic Society guidelines for the management of community-acquired pneumonia in children: <www.brit-thoracic. org.uk>.

CHAPTER 8: ABDOMINAL PAIN
eMedicine health, 'Abdominal pain in children': <www. emedicinehealth.com/abdominal_pain_in_children/article_ em.htm>
MedicineNet.com: <medicinenet.com/colic/index.htm>.
Patient UK, 'Recurrent abdominal pain in children': <www.patient. co.uk/showdoc/40002007/>.

CHAPTER 9: VOMITING AND DIARRHOEA

Dehydration table adapted from World Health Organization, *The Treatment of Diarrhoea*, 4th revision, 2005.

A Levine, KA Santaucci, DW Marby, 'Paediatrics, Gastroenteritis': <www.emedicine.com/EMERG/topic380.htm>.

DM D'Alessandro, 'Acute Abdominal Pain Through the Ages': <www.pediatriceducation.org/2005/09/19>.

EJ Elliott, 'Acute Gastroenteritis in Children', *BMJ*, 334, pp. 35–40, 6 January 2007.

CHAPTER 17: INJURY PREVENTION

JG Berry, JE Harrison, *Hospital separations due to Injury and Poisoning, Australia 2003–04*, AIHW, Canberra, 2007.

The Swimming Pools Act 1992: <www.dlg.nsw.gov.au>.

CHAPTER 21: BITES AND STINGS

International Liaison Committee on Resuscitation 2005 Consensus on ECC & CPR Science and Treatment Recommendations, 'Worksheet First Aid – What is the safety, efficacy and feasibility of compressive wrapping for coral snake (elapid) envenomation'.

CHAPTER 23: THE 'SAFE' APPROACH

Australian Resuscitation Council, 'Guidelines': <www.resus.org.au>.

'The 1998 European Resuscitation Council guidelines for adult single rescuer basic life support', *BMJ*, 316: 1870–76, 20 June 1998.

CHAPTER 24: BASIC LIFE SUPPORT

International Liaison Committee on Resuscitation, '2005 International Consensus Conference on Cardiopulmonary Resuscitation and Emergency Cardiovascular Care Science With Treatment Recommendations', *Circulation*, 112(suppl), pp. 73–90, 2005.

——'2005 International Consensus Conference on Cardiopulmonary Resuscitation and Emergency Cardiovascular Care Science With Treatment Recommendations', *Resuscitation*, 67, pp. 271–91, 2005.

Australian Resuscitation Council, 'Guidelines for Resuscitation', March 2006: <www.resus.org.au>.

INDEX

PHOTO CREDITS

The publishers would like to thank the following for the use of their photographs:

iStockphoto: pp 82, 145, 185, 191

Photolibrary: pp 146 (l), 148 (all)

Custom Medical Stock Photo: p 149 (r)

Dr Pam Brown: p 150

Mediscan: p 151

Mr James W Fairley, Consultant ENT Surgeon, Kent, UK,
<www.entkent.com>: p 157

Getty Photos: p 216

Flagstaff photos: pp 225 (all), 228

Commonwealth of Australia/GBRMPA: p 232 (l above, l & r below)

Dr Jamie Seymour: p 232 (r above)

Shutterstock: p 241